W9-ADQ-620

RHINOPLASTY: EMPHASIZING THE EXTERNAL APPROACH

Published volumes

Proportions of the Aesthetic Face
Powell & Humphreys
Facial Reconstruction with Local and Regional Flaps
Becker

The American Academy of Facial Plastic and Reconstructive Surgery

Series Editor: James D. Smith, M.D.

RHINOPLASTY: EMPHASIZING THE EXTERNAL APPROACH

Jack R. Anderson, M.D.
Clinical Professor, Departments of
   Otolaryngology: Head and Neck Surgery
Louisiana State University Medical School
Tulane University Medical School
New Orleans, Louisiana

W. Russell Ries, M.D.
Nashville, Tennessee

1986
Thieme Inc., New York
Georg Thieme Verlag   Stuttgart • New York

Thieme Inc.
381 Park Avenue South
New York, New York 10016

Series sponsored by the educational committee of The American Academy of Facial Plastic and Reconstructive Surgery.

Library of Congress Cataloging in Publication Data
Anderson, Jack R., 1917–
    Rhinoplasty : emphasizing the external approach.

(The American Academy of Facial Plastic and Reconstructive Surgery)
    Bibliography: p.
    Includes index.
    1. Rhinoplasty. I. Ries, W. Russell, 1953–
II. Title. III. Series: The American Academy of Facial
Plastic and Reconstructive Surgery (Series) [DNLM:
1. Rhinoplasty—methods. WV 312 A547r]
RF350.A53   1986   617'.523   86-14424
ISBN 0-86577-238-X

Cover design by M. Losaw

Printed in the United States of America

RHINOPLASTY: EMPHASIZING THE
EXTERNAL APPROACH
Anderson and Ries

0-85677-238-X (Thieme Inc.)
3-13-691501-1 (Georg Thieme Verlag)

0-86577-137-5 (series)
3-13-656501-0 (series)

5 4 3 2 1

Contents

17. Secondary Rhinoplasty   113

18. Chin Augmentation   123

19. Case Discussions   125

    References   172

    Index   175

Preface

The stimulus for writing this volume was the passing of a colleague I had known for many years. He was a New Yorker, and New York was the mecca of the rhinoplasty world 35 years ago, when we first met. I thought my friend was doing the best rhinoplasties in New York at that time, even though others I had visited were more renowned; he was, even then, using columella struts, shield grafts and other types of artistry that are considered the latest advances today.

The trouble was, he was not a good communicator. He wrote but little, and he was not a good speaker. All his knowledge was locked in his head. Several times during his later years, I told him that we ought to get together and talk about rhinoplasty while a tape recorder was running—my hope was, of course, that I could edit his remarks so that some of his vast knowledge could be passed on. Alas, we never got around to doing that, and his wisdom has been lost forever.

I am sure that I do not know as much as my friend knew, nor am I as surgically expert as he was. But I have learned a number of useful things from him and others during the past 35 years and do not want to repeat his mistake of not passing them on. Perhaps they will help others avoid some of the mistakes I made along the way because I firmly subscribe to the adage "The smart man learns from the mistakes of others, the fool must learn from his own mistakes."

Being, by nature, an improver rather than an innovator, I must confess that there is little really new in this volume. The notions presented have evolved from watching many rhinoplasty surgeons work, reading articles they wrote and listening to them speak at meetings and courses. Stored in my CPR, they were subsequently modified for my purposes. In the process, their origins have been obliterated by the passage of time in many instances, so few specific references have been introduced into the body of the text. Rather, a general bibliography is provided. I hope that the failure to cite sources will be understood and the omission forgiven.

Something that should be interesting to newcomers to the field of rhinoplasty is that the external approach to the operation is emphasized. The wide exposure it provides permits greater accuracy and control and enables a dedicated surgeon to become experienced and skilled much quicker than otherwise.

Finally, it is customary to thank everyone connected with the production of such a monograph, and my co-author and I will not act to the contrary. We thank our families and our friends for their encouragement. We thank the members of our office and hospital staffs whom we feel work with us, not for us. We thank all those surgeons who passed their knowledge on to us over the years in lectures, in the medical literature, in demonstrations, and also in informal conversations. Our thanks go to those whom we have taught, our Residents and Fellows and those who have attended our courses and lectures; it has often been said that teachers often learn more than their students—that is so true! In a very special way, we thank our patients, for each of them offered us a new opportunity to learn.

Very special appreciation goes to Eugene New who did most of the illustrations. He was very understanding and cooperative, as was Mr. Felix Schillesci, our medical photographer for the past 35 years.

Special thanks also go to The American Academy of Facial Plastic and Reconstructive Surgery for asking us to write the monograph. We have tried to justify their expression of confidence and hope the contents will meet their educational objectives.

Jack R. Anderson, M.D.
New Orleans, 1986

Introduction

Rhinoplastic surgery may be either cosmetic or reconstructive. The purpose of cosmetic rhinoplasty, the subject of this book, is to enhance the appearance of a nose which, though not perfect, falls within the range of general acceptability. Reconstructive rhinoplasty, on the other hand, usually implies tissue deficit from trauma or disease, and is performed to try to restore both function and appearance to as near normal as possible.

The basic concept of rhinoplasty seems simple enough at first glance: one removes the nasal hump, shortens and narrows the nose, and then remodels the tip. Yet, things are not always what they seem. Many surgeons, including eminently experienced ones, have run aground during the operation, thereby confirming the old adage, "There's nothing so complicated as simplicity."

Actually rhinoplasty is a complex and demanding procedure, perhaps moreso than most other cosmetic operations. For example, we once engaged a medical photographer to photograph all the surgical steps of a moderately difficult septorhinoplasty and ended up with 134 Kodachrome slides! In addition, the nose is like a signpost for everyone to see since it is the most prominent feature of the face. Therefore results that might be acceptable in an area of the body hidden from public view could be unwelcome after cosmetic surgery of the nose.

It is a thinking surgeon's operation. Besides surgical ability, it requires extreme accuracy and infinite attention to detail. It cannot be performed by rote because each nose presents a different set of problems, and the changes projected are usually only in terms of millimeters. Furthermore, some of the surgical steps create deformities that must, in turn, be corrected. At the conclusion, all of the pieces must fit into place like a jig-saw puzzle to produce the final picture. As if this were not enough, allowance must be made for changes that invariably occur during healing. All of this is in addition to the basic need for sound diagnosis and an appreciation of both aesthetic principles and the limiting factors in a given case.

There are more psychologic implications than in many other types of surgery. Yet, cosmetic surgeons have only a relatively short time to uncover the true motivations and expectations of prospective patients and to determine if they have sufficient ego-strength to cope with the operation and its results; that is why cosmetic surgeons sometimes humorously refer to themselves as "thirty-minute psychiatrists."

And, medicolegal exposure for rhinoplasty surgeons is greater than for most other physicians. Despite the fact that the changes patients request are often only in terms of millimeters, surgeons are being held to higher and higher standards as the public becomes more sophisticated and attorneys become more rapacious.

An immutable truth emerges: the criterion for success in any cosmetic surgery is a satisfied patient, not necessarily a satisfied doctor. Fortunately, most patients are pleased with less than their surgeons are, but some are dissatisfied even with good results, especially if they don't obtain the validation they expected from others. That is why surgeons should establish and adhere to stringent criteria for patient acceptance, why one must be careful not to operate badly, and why the practice of good interpersonal relations is so important.

In spite of all these impediments, the practice of rhinoplastic surgery has much to offer a physician, particularly if he is challenged by opportunity, willing to work hard and enjoys work situations in which he gets fairly rapid and concrete feedback on how he is doing. It is especially attractive to achievement-oriented people, which most successful cosmetic surgeons are, because of their penchant for spending a great deal of time thinking about ways to improve things or do them better.

Reconstructive rhinoplasty has been performed for several centuries, but it is understandable that rhinoplasty for purely aesthetic purposes could not gain widespread acceptance until a technique was developed to eliminate external scarring. This was first reported by Roe, an otolaryngologist of Rochester, New York in 1891; he described a technique whereby the entire operation could be performed via an endonasal approach.

Other small contributions were made after that, but Jacques Joseph, an orthopedist of Berlin, Germany must be acknowledged to be the father of cosmetic rhinoplasty. He probed the causes of nasal deformities, ingeniously devised means and instruments to correct them surgically, and in 1928 published a report of his experiences in a monumental volume entitled "Nasenplastick und Sontige Gesichtsplastic Nebst Mammoplastik."

The surgical dynamics of the operation as established by Joseph remain unchanged. However, as time passed and surgeons and their patients became more sophisticated, results were submitted to more critical scrutiny. This led to the developments of technical variations and refinements for solving specific problems and achieving certain goals.

The senior author's study of rhinoplasty began in 1952 with exposure to Fomon, who must be credited with kindling the interest of otolaryngologists in the operation, even though he wasn't an otolaryngologist himself.

Subsequently, we have associated with most of the leading surgeons of the era and learned from them. We have taught thousands in courses sponsored by the American Academy of Facial Plastic and Reconstructive Surgery, the American Academy of Otolaryngology: Head and Neck Surgery, Tulane and other universities and learned from them. Finally, we have performed an estimated 7000 to 8000 rhinoplasties and have learned from them. So, ours is an eclectic approach.

We certainly do not claim that our methods are the best nor that they are the only ones available to solve the problems one faces in practice; they are the ones we have found useful. We still change them in minor ways from time to time as we discover things that will improve results, make life easier, and render better service to patients. We do, however, have a good reason for everything we do or do not do based on our past experience. Since we are firm advocates of the eclectic approach to the practice of this type of surgery, we sincerely hope that the reader will find a few things appealing enough to incorporate into his regimen of patient management.

As previously intimated, we believe that true success in rhinoplasty, or in any other type of cosmetic surgery, does not stem from technical expertise only; a number of other elements are important, too. Above all, one must be dedicated and enthusiastic, practice good interpersonal relations and continuously study his results for the purpose of improvement.

A surgeon need not be an artist, as some would have the public believe, nor does he have to possess a rare and unique talent. He should attempt to become a good artisan who understands the material with which he works and tries to develop a sense of balance, symmetry and appropriateness. Furthermore, he need not operate brilliantly on every occasion, but he should not operate badly, two quite different things. He must try to understand what is causing the deformity he seeks to correct and know a number of different surgical techniques so that he can effectively cope with any eventualities that might arise. He should be appropriately supportive of the patient during the postoperative period. Finally, he must recognize his own limitations, for it is equally important to know when he should and should not operate.

When one has acquired the ability to satisfy capably all the special demands or requirements of a particular situation, craft or profession, he is generally said to be competent; neither operating speed or personal publicity should ever be confused with competence. It should be pointed out that finishing a residency program or passing a board examination indicates that a small segment of a surgeon's peers believe he has learned enough to operate safely on his own. This is, however, only the beginning of a long process of self-education aimed at developing competence. There are no short cuts, just as there are no short cuts to quality. Therein lies the reason cosmetic facial surgery, particularly rhinoplasty, is so demanding a mistress.

1　Appearance: Cultural and Social Considerations

An important feature of man's cultural development has been his inclination to bring beauty into his environment. Some, like artists of various types, try to create it; the remainder try to possess it in one way or the other — in the selection of what we buy, how we dress, how we groom ourselves, how we beautify our surroundings, and, even how we select our friends and mates. This need to create or possess beauty seems to have become so ingrained that it might almost be termed an instinct.

The microcosm that is cosmetic surgery mirrors the larger movement; the surgeon has the urge to develop beauty or, at least, to improve the surroundings, whereas his patients want to possess something better than what they have. This is why it would be well for each rhinoplastic surgeon, at some point in his career, to delve into the philosophic foundation underlying his calling.

WHAT IS BEAUTY?

Logically speaking, the first question to be asked is, "What is beauty?" Defining beauty, like defining love, is well-nigh impossible, but a useful definition might be that it is whatever is pleasing or attractive to the senses, mainly to the eye in the context of our discussion.

Most persons are conformists and seem to agree surprisingly well on who is beautiful; their concepts depend on the taste of the times, the culture, and their ethnic derivations. Furthermore, our tastes today, like it or not, are influenced to a large extent by television, motion pictures, the media, and the public relations industry; the danger is that these entities will cause taste to become more standardized and, thus, more monotonous in the future.

To be sure, the concept of beauty changes over the years; but, if one studies faces that are generally considered to be beautiful, the one element that seems to be constant is the harmonious relationship of the features to each other and to the whole. In other words, good proportion, a comparative relationship between the parts, exists.

There are other components of beauty, of course, such as the color values and textures of the skin, facial expressions (of which there are said to be more than 250,000), and the ease and grace of facial movements. However, one thing is certain: no face can be considered beautiful if there is distortion and inappropriateness of features.

THE IMPORTANCE OF APPEARANCE

Appearance is important in our culture because it affects how others react to us and how we feel about ourselves. Most people learn early in life that ugliness is a stigma that triggers discrimination, and this knowledge is reinforced continuously. As a matter of fact, most of us have been guilty of such prejudice at times.

Psychosocial studies have confirmed these premises on many occasions; for example, it has been shown that:

1. Six-year-old children react differently to their attractive and unattractive peers.
2. Teachers often think that unattractive children have less intellectual, educational, and athletic potential; they are, also, more likely to describe them as maladjusted and antisocial when they misbehave.
3. Good-looking people are thought to be kinder, more interesting, warmer, more poised and self-assertive, more successful, more competent as lovers or spouses, and happier, in general, then unattractive individuals.
4. Nice-looking waitresses earn more than double the tips of homely ones.
5. Juries tend to go easier on attractive defendants; they acquit them more often and give them lighter sentences when convicted.
6. Employment agencies frequently rate people on good-looks and deportment as well as their qualifications.

7. Attractive applicants for lower level jobs are hired more often and receive higher starting pay than plainer ones.

8. Less attractive patients in psychiatric hospitals have more severe diagnoses, are hospitalized for longer periods, get less attention from attendants, and have fewer visitors. Incidentally, it is well-known that increased interest in personal appearance is one of the first changes that occurs when a person is emerging from a psychotic episode.

Our bias against unattractiveness is reinforced by another cultural defect — we are prone to take outward signs as a reflection of the type of person an individual is. The "image makers" of Hollywood, the political arena, and industry work on this premise: they "package" people so that they are favorably received by the targeted audience. For example, the appearance of youth is equated with vigor, creativity, and the ability to function, whereas the older person is presented as being set in his ways, past his prime, and on the downgrade. The reverse of this might also be used, as occurred during the 1980 presidential campaign. Reacting to charges that Ronald Reagen was too old to assume the office of President, he was shown bared to the waist chopping wood at his ranch and riding horses, and the public was convinced otherwise. Likewise, neat people are thought of as being interested in or thinking well of themselves; therefore, the usual view is that this characteristic will carry over into their jobs and personal lives.

The bottom line therefore is that appearance shapes judgment about character, status, social acceptability, and potential achievement. Another truism is that first impressions are especially important in our society.

Peculiar interactional dynamics are set in motion when two individuals meet for the first time. Since faces are usually the center of attention in the beginning, their physical characteristics and features are the only things available to grab hold of. If we are favorably impressed, first impressions can color every subsequent judgment we make; if unfavorable, they may, in like manner, prejudice all of our succeeding estimates of a person's merit.

Incidentally, it has been shown that when strangers meet, whether it be socially, professionally, or, even, in some levels of the job market, the first 4 minutes or so are the most important of the encounter. During that time, they are each looking for clues to formulate a judgment as to whether to continue the relationship further or to pass on. Some even experience immediate feelings of like or dislike during that brief interval.

Such rapid categorization of people on the basis of first impressions can lead to uncritical and erroneous estimates that operate to the disadvantage of those whose features are unpleasant or deformed in any way. This may be irrational, but it does exist, and people know this. This is one reason why most consider grooming and appearance to be so important. They want to be admired for qualities that they either have or can simulate.

THE *PSYCHOLOGY TODAY* SURVEY

Some appreciation of the extent of appearance concern in American life can be gleaned from the results of a body image survey conducted during 1972 and 1973 by the popular magazine *Psychology Today*. There were 62,000 readers, a sizeable sample, who returned a 109 item body image questionnaire with the following results:

20 percent (50 million Americans) did not like their nose

12 percent (30 million) did not like their chins

6 percent (5 million) did not like their eyes

6 percent did not like their ears

20 percent did not like their hair (or lack of it)

25 percent (62 million) did not like their complexion

There were a number of other revelations that should interest cosmetic surgeons or those entering the field. Both men and women agreed nearly equally that physical attractiveness is very important in day-to-day social interaction for most people. Women are generally less satisfied with their body image than men are. Their dissatisfaction persists and remains stable as they age, perhaps because more beauty bias is directed against women in our society.

Body image is only one component of self-esteem, for persons who are satisfied with their faces are more self-confident; they feel themselves to be more likable, assertive, conscientious, and even more intelligent than the "average person."

The preadolescent years are critical in the development of one's body image, and teasing in early life has a lasting effect. Men and women who felt homely as children tend to be less satisfied with their bodies as adults. The unattractive child or teenager is often miserable and remembers that misery throughout life. However, sudden changes in appearance can be stressful, even if for the better, and do not guarantee happiness. Multiple changers are less happy, less self-confident, and have worse body images than those who change once or never.

In concluding their report on the results of the survey, the authors wrote:

> "George Bernard Shaw once noted that "beauty is all very well, but who ever looks at it when it has been in the house three days?" The answer is, almost everybody.
>
> Our respondents strongly agreed that physical attractiveness is important in getting along with others, in acquiring mates, in having good sex lives, in feeling satisfied with themselves. Good looks were important to respondents from small towns and large cities, to people who have travelled widely and those who have stayed home, to people who deal constantly with strangers and those who work with friends.

Personality and self-esteem do not rest exclusively on satisfaction with one's body, but neither is the body an irrelevant shell in which the soul happens to live. We treat beautiful people differently from the way we treat homely ones, and denying this truth will not make a person's looks less important.

Some *Psychology Today* readers have escaped the tyranny of attractiveness, but others admit they never will: "I am 30 years old, a success in a field few women enter, a good speaker, conversationalist, and clown,...I am happily married and feel valued by my family, but I'd chuck it all if some Mephistophelean character offered me the option of the kind of long-legged, acquiline, tawny beauty praised in myth and toothpaste ads."

OPTIONS

When a person becomes dissatisfied with the appearance of a particular feature, he has, roughly, four options available to make him content:

1. He may downgrade its importance and compensate by developing the other components of self-esteem (such as learning, success, talent, personality, and charm).
2. He can resort to camouflage or enhancement by dress and grooming, among others.

3. If he is expending too much psychic energy on the problem, he can seek psychiatric care in an attempt to change his attidue.
4. He may try to rid himself of his preoccupation by resorting to cosmetic surgery if the deformity is, indeed, amendable to correction.

DISCUSSION

Our culture is not a substitute for the past; it is a link with it. As early as the dawn of Western civilization, the hallmarks of beauty had been estblished, and they have had their effect on human relations through the ensuing centuries.

Today, however, because of our highly sophisticated methods of communication, more persons seem to be more appearance-conscious than ever before. We have been urged so frequently by advertisements in every medium to improve our appearance that it has almost become a duty and responsibility to use every method possible to do so. Although it is true that a pleasing appearance is certainly no substitute for ability, lack of it may close the door initially to many opportunities.

As a result of this "brainwashing" and because ours has become a competitive, youth-oriented world, Americans spend upwards of $20 billion a year and a great deal of time and effort on their faces and bodies, largely to make a good impression, to win approval, and to bring them happiness. Things that were considered evidence of vanity or luxury at one time are now considered necessary for business, social, and emotional reasons.

It is unlikely that society will change and that appearance will ever become less important to the majority of people. This may seem superficial to some, but it obviously results from strong social and cultural currents.

Nor should it be mistakenly attributed to vanity. A large component of vanity is a desire to excel over one's fellow man. Our experience has been that most patients interested in having appearance surgery want just the opposite; they want to conform to current standards.

2 Cosmetic Surgeon: Image, Appearance, and Environment

Building a successful cosmetic surgery practice does not depend solely on technical competence; mostly, it depends on the surgeon's personality and his understanding of the milieu in which he functions. Like it or not, he is rendering a service to the public in the medical marketplace. So, besides doing good work, which many others also do, he must develop a pleasing personality and sell himself and his product ethically.

The concept of salesmanship in medicine may be anathematic to some, but it is a fact of life. Salesmanship is a key part of the free enterprise system; everyone is selling something: himself, his talent, a product, an idea, even a way of life. A fundamental fact every salesman knows is that prospects buy the impression he creates as much as the service he provides, so it behooves those who would like to develop busy practices to give some attention to this aspect of their professional lives.

PERSONALITY

Wright surveyed a number of successful cosmetic surgeons in order to construct a profile of their personalities. Her sampling indicated that they have increased needs to achieve, excel, control, be seen in a favorable light, are defensive when faced with a psychologic threat, and, finally, their expectations usually exceed those of their patients. To these might be added enthusiasm, optimism, a sensitivity to disproportion in facial structure, a zeal to create beauty (the Pygmalion complex), and a desire to help people (the Savior complex).

Feedback from their practices sometimes has an extraordinary effect on the personalities of cosmetic surgeons. Other physicians spend a good deal of time trying to relieve pain and suffering and frequently can make only a small difference in the outcome of a disease, whereas the cosmetic surgeon works under conditions that seem to be almost ideal. First, the patients are well; secondly, unlike others, they want the operations, so they usually do well postoperatively; and, lastly, 85 percent are satisfied with the results in the long run.

This milieu of success results in a great deal of adulation being heaped on the surgeon by patients and society in general. If he substitutes the judgment of the public for that of his more knowledgeable peers, the very real danger exists that he will begin to believe his own "press notices" and develop an inflated sense of importance and omniscience. This can be destructuve from the standpoint of both the surgeon and the public, for no mortal can always operate brilliantly; rather, the goal should be not to operate badly.

Wright has also pointed out that the very factors that make the cosmetic surgeon's work extremely satisfactory often make it difficult for him to accept the dissatisfied patient. Thus, the surgeon must be very careful to maintain his sensitivity to his patient's emotional needs, not only when things are going well, but, also, when they go wrong.

Guze has noted how ironic it is that the very patients who should be entitled to a full measure of compassion, since they continue to suffer because they are not helped, are the ones we tend to treat with the least understanding and sympathy. Some cosmetic surgeons prefer to avoid such patients, disparage them if they complain, blame them for their troubles, and act as though they feel that the patients really do not appreciate the efforts expended to help them.

Part of this results from the dichotomy of viewpoints toward cosmetic surgery. The patient views it only in an esthetic way and thinks in terms of the effects it has on him, especially the sensations it stimulates and the feeling it elicits. The surgeon's viewpoint is both aesthetic and artistic; he thinks in terms of technique, the relationship of the details to the whole, and the effects to be achieved with what he has to work with. In essence, he regards success as a thing that results from attention to these matters. Common to both viewpoints, however, is a desire for perfection associated with one's conception of an ideal.

Nonetheless, it should not be forgotten that a cosmetic surgeon's ultimate success depends on whether or not his patients are pleased, not whether he is pleased.

CATEGORIZING THE COSMETIC SURGEON

There are abundant implications in both the medical and lay press that the cosmetic surgeon is an "artist," the suggestion being that he has been given or possesses some special talent that sets him apart, but is he an artist?

Strictly speaking, an artist is one who does anything well, with a feeling for form and effect. Creativity is implied. Related categories include: "artisans," whose work is mechanical and who are skilled workmen; "artificers," who come between artists and artisans in that they put more constructive thought, skill, intelligence, and taste into their work than do artisans, but less of the idealizing power than do artists; and, finally, "mechanics," who construct anything by mere routine and rule.

If one subscribes to the purest idea that creation involves bringing something into existence out of nothing, then the cosmetic surgeon is, of course, not an artist, as is sometimes described in the puffery of the media. He may, however, become a finished practitioner in his occupation, which, indisputably, requires skill that can be acquired by study, training, and experience.

IMAGE, APPEARANCE, AND BEHAVIOR

It should be remembered that patients come to a cosmetic surgeon's office with preconceived images formed as a result of the exposure to television, the movies, the lay media, and other patients. Sometimes, these images are erroneous and may have to be dispelled; on the other hand, they are sometimes accurate, and surgeons have to live up to them when they are.

Related to this is the fact that there is a strong human tendency to see things in emotionally consistent ways; for example, bad people usually cannot be expected to engage in a good act. Therefore, how a patient perceives a doctor sometimes has a remarkable effect on the patient's psychology. If he is won over by the doctor's personality, character, attitude, personal motives, and interest in him as an individual, he will consider it an honor to be associated with him, and understanding, cooperation, and good will flow from this.

Some desirable characteristics in a cosmetic surgeon include friendliness and interest in the patient, not just in signing him up for an operation. One way of demonstrating this early in the relationship is by conducting an unhurried consultation during which a good history is taken, a factual explanation offered as to what is involved in the procedure requested, including the limitations, and the patient's questions are answered truthfully, without evasiveness.

Since patients generally admire professionals who give the impression that they know what they are talking about, vacillation can be destructive to the relationship. However, although one should project the image of being self-assured and authoritative, any semblance of cockiness should be avoided; in particular, one should keep clear of any careless remarks that might imply a warranty.

A surgeon should establish the ground rules of the relationship early and remain in control. He should not succumb to flattery nor allow the patient to endow him with omnipotence ("Doctor, make me beautiful," or "I'll leave everything in your hands; do whatever you think."). Furthermore, he should not let the patient become manipulative, that is, change his routine or fee policy, rush things, or try to engage him in duplicity to secure insurance reimbursement when none is indicated. The best way we have found to handle such situations is to tell the patient that these things engender in us a feeling of "dys-ease," and we cannot do our best work when we are upset.

On the other hand, the surgeon should not become antagonistic if the patient disagrees with his assessment and recommendations; that is, certainly, the patient's privilege. Conversely, of course, one should never be persuaded to proceed with any operation he feels is not in the best interest of the patient or himself.

Finally, an eagerness to operate seems to be one of the hallmarks of cosmetic surgeons; this is due mainly, perhaps, to the satisfaction they derive from plying their craft. It begins during their training, carries over into the practice-building phase, and later segues into the period when the practice is firmly established. However, it is terribly important not to give the patient the impression that he is being "sold" the surgery. This is not only inconsistent with our professional obligations and responsibilities, but it may also upset the patient, cause him to become defensive, and engender the feeling that the surgeon's interest in him is mainly pecuniary. Then, too, if a "hustled" patient becomes dissatisfied with the results of an operation, the onus must be borne entirely by the surgeon.

CLOTHES AND APPEARANCE

Important parts of a cosmetic surgeon's image and appearance are his grooming and his dress; these things, as well as his environment, making a strong personal statement. Some regard clothes as only something to cover one's skin; at the other extreme are those who use clothes to allow them to imitate a peacock. On the other hand, they can be used to subliminally project the image of authority, power, success, and influence and to give confidence and engender it in others.

The research of Molloy, whom *Time* magazine has called "a wardrobe engineer," indicates that conservative class-conscious conformity, as far as clothes are concerned, is absolutely essential to the individual business and professional man. His surveys revealed that what matters about a person's dress and hairstyle is not what the individual thinks about it himself, or what society in general thinks about it. What matters is the opinion of those who are in a position to make judgments that will either help or hurt; in our context, these are our patients.

Since most of the patients in a cosmetic surgical practice usually come from the middle or upper middle class, we should strongly consider conforming to their general average of dress rather than otherwise; for example, practicing in an open neck sport shirt with a gold chain and medallion around one's neck would be inappropriate in most parts of the country, and even in many parts of California. Therefore, a surgeon's clothes should be appropriate; what might be fitting for the beach or a sporting event would be unseemly in the office, at the hospital, or at medical meetings.

The clothes need not be expensive, but they should look expensive without being ostentatious. Someone has said of clothes that, like old money, they should whisper, "not shout"; putting it another way, they should be quietly elegant, and the color range should be subdued.

Finally, a necktie is always good form, even when one is casually attired in a blazer.

OFFICE ENVIRONMENT

Having been preconditioned by the media, most persons who consult a cosmetic surgeon expect that his office will be more attractive and less clinical looking than the usual doctor's office. Although a good-looking office and dressing well will not enhance a surgeon's ability, they are important from the standpoint of the initial impression they make on the patient. Bare, drab offices affect patients in a negative way and cause them unconsciously to question the stature and up-to-date knowledge of their owners; on the other hand, attractive surroundings project an image of success and provide an emotional uplift, not only for the patient but, more importantly, for the surgeon and his staff. Going "first class" and knowing it is "the best" can be a tremendous boost for self-confidence and enthusiasm.

Most large corporations appreciate the fact that environment plays an important part in the mood and feeling of their employees and customers, so they hire industrial designers to use light, color, and form expertly to improve their surroundings and image. This same approach can be used by physicians to a lesser degree.

The appearance of the reception room is most important. An initial positive image establishes the relationship on a proper footing by helping to allay any apprehension the patient may have and, also, serves to build the patient's confidence in the doctor. Toward that end, it should be furnished like a living room in one's home; the carpets, wall coverings, furnishings, and accessories should all be color coordinated; the lighting should be indirect or provided by lamps; magazines should be current; the use of soft background music might be considered. If the room is small, mirroring one wall will create an illusion of depth. Any art works hanging on the wall should be carefully chosen and appropriately framed to match the decor. Finally, it is important that the patient's waiting area should not be open to the working area of the receptionist.

This same homelike motif should be carried throughout the office, if possible. Halls should be wide and carpeted to minimize noise, since they are apt to be the most highly trafficked areas.

It is well to set aside one or more private consultation rooms that are devoted exclusively to conferring with new patients or with persons who have not yet decided to have surgery. Again, they should be elegantly decorated and furnished to establish an informal, luxurious, nonclinical atmosphere, designed to put the patient at ease and inspire confidence.

Ideally, the office should be "zoned" around a receptionist-business office core that services the zones. One zone consists of the consultation rooms and the other includes the treatment rooms and the office surgical suite serviced by a nurses' station; between the two zones, in addition to the receptionist-business office core, it is useful also to have an inner waiting room and a room that can be used for photography and postoperative cosmetology.

OFFICE STAFF

The importance of one's office staff in a cosmetic surgery practice cannot be overestimated. In many ways they are the practice because they represent the office everytime they answer the telephone, deal with a patient, or deal with the public. The mind-set of a potential patient, a new patient, or an old patient can definitely be affected by the reaction to the staff. The pleasant attitude and solicitous cooperation of everyone in the office help paint the mental picture an outsider gets from a doctor's organization. Friendly people make a friendly office, the kind that is a real pleasure to deal with, so each employee should consider himself or herself an "ambassador of goodwill."

Thus, members of the staff should be carefully chosen. Besides being competent and efficient, they should like people, be friendly, and be made to feel that they are working with the surgeon, not for him. They should be painstakingly educated about all the aspects of cosmetic surgery so that they know what the surgeon is trying to accomplish; then they can be imaginative in helping him achieve that objective. Their conduct may be informal and friendly, but it should always be decorous; they should never speak about other patients or disparage the work of other surgeons.

Because some patients are more inclined to reveal to members of the office staff their fears, hopes, and any untoward incidents they have experienced than to the surgeon, staff members should report any pertinent facts they glean while alone with the patient because such data can often facilitate patient management.

Finally, everyone reacts favorably to "stroking," and this includes members of one's staff. They should be praised from time to time for their efforts, loayalty, and dedication; they should be thanked for their pleasantness, patience, and willingness to do more than their job description calls for — to go that one step further. In this connection, it is better to praise the act than the person, for that doubles the impact, reinforces sincerity, and creates an incentive for more of the same. Finally, it is better to thank people when they least expect it; this shows sensitivity and consideration for other people and strengthens loyalty.

3   Medicolegal Aspects

Each time a physician treats a patient, whether it be for the first time or on a return visit, the possibility of a malpractice suit exists. It is humanly impossible to eliminate all legal risks. However, they can be minimized by learning one's legal obligations to patients, by foreseeing probable hazards, and by exercising good professional judgment and discretion. Whatever legal risks remain after that, the physician must accept if he wants to continue practicing medicine.

Being sued for medical malpractice is a very traumatic experience, emotionally; it affects not only a physician's personal and social life, but also it changes one's manner of practice, and even philosophy.

Malpractice suits have become more common for several reasons. Today, unlike former times, people are more likely to resort to legal action whenever they think, however erroneously, that someone else has done something that interferes with their rights and privileges. This tendency is aided and abetted by some attorneys, who exploit the situation, and by the news media, which gives the public a distorted view of the value of personal injury claims by prominently reporting large demands initially but giving the matter little or no attention later if the action results in a judgment in favor of the physician or if the award is for a conservative amount. Finally, courts and juries are now holding physicians to a higher degree of responsibility than ever before. All this, of course, adds to the cost of medical care.

Those who seek cosmetic surgery freuqently have some neurotic overlay. Since success in cosmetic surgery is measured by the patient's, not the physician's, satisfaction, patients are likely candidates for filing a suit if anything goes wrong, if they do not like the result, or if the result does not live up to their expectations.

This is why cosmetic surgeons are put in one of the highest risk classifications for medical liability insurance. High risk means that physicians in that class generate claims that produce a high total cost to the company; either the average cost of the claims is high, or the frequency is high, or both the cost and frequency are high. Even un-successful claims can cost a company money for legal fees, for expert witnesses, for investigation, and for general administrative expenses.

We do not believe that all malpractice actions are unjustified, nor that it is wrong to hold physicians in their professional lives to the standards they are held in their private lives as members of society; as a matter of fact, we think that an appreciation of their legal risks can cause physicians to practice better medicine. Some patients should be compensated, and some physicians should be sued. The bottom line is that the best practice medically is usually the best practice legally; nowhere is the Golden Rule more applicable.

THE PHYSICIAN AND THE LAW

Like any other citizen, a physician may run afoul of the law in two large areas:

1. Criminal law: when he does something that is inimical to the interests of society as a whole (State vs. Person)
2. Civil law: when he is sued by another person to obtain personal compensation or some other type of redress for a wrong he has done (Person vs. Person; torts)

Because a contract is established each time a physician accepts a patient for treatment, he may also be sued for breach of contract if he promises favorable results that do not occur — the courts hold that a patient has the right to rely on what his physician tells him. It should be noted, however, that mere disappointment with the results of an operation is not grounds for recovery against a surgeon, unless the surgeon had specifically guaranteed a particular result that was not forthcoming.

The two torts of which physicians are most frequently accused are: (1) the treatment rendered was not authorized by the patient; and (2) the patient was harmed by treatment that did not measure up to professional standards. The first is legally known as "battery" and the second is labeled "negligence" or "malpractice."

The burden of proof in any professional liability suit is on the patient who brings the suit, except when the doctrine of "res ipse loquitur" is invoked; then the courts and juries assume the defendent physician to be guilty until he proves he was not negligent.

THE PHYSICIAN - PATIENT CONTRACT

Contracts may be written, oral, or implied; the latter two types are the most usual ones that are established between the doctor and his patient. Not everyone is legally competent to enter into a contract, and payment is not essential for such a contract to be binding. The contract exists even if the patient is not being charged by the physician.

The terms of the contract imposed by law create more obligations on the physician than on the patient; among these are:

1. He must not take advantage of the patient in any way, such as operate without the patient's informed consent.
2. He may not withhold information necessary for the patient's health or welfare.
3. He may not disclose information about the patient to others without the patient's written consent (invasion of privacy).
4. Once he has accepted the patient for treatment, his obligation is a continuing one, as long as the need for continuing medical care exists.
5. He can end the relationship only by giving advance notice that allows the patient reasonable time to obtain the services of another physician.
6. He must possess that degree of skill ordinarily possessed by physicians of his professional status in similar circumstances, regardless of locale if he professes to be a specialist, and he is expected to exercise that skill in the care of his patient.
7. He must adequately supervise any aspects of the patient's medical care that he delegates to others.
8. He must not give an expressed or im-

plied warranty regarding the success of any treatment he renders.

On the other hand, the patient is obligated not to withhold information the physician needs for proper conduct of treatment, and he must agree to follow the physician's instructions. Finally, the physician may withdraw from the case provided he gives the patient proper and timely notification and continues treatment until the patient selects a replacement.

BATTERY AND INFORMED CONSENT

The law holds that, since it is the patient's body, he has the right to decide what to do with it. Therefore a surgical procedure done without advance consent, whether expressed or implied, is "battery" or "trespass" in the legal sense, and the surgeon becomes liable even if his intent was good, or, in fact, if his intent was to do no harm. The patient need not prove actual injury, only that his rights were violated. The courts have said, in effect, that because a good doctor will inform his patients of the risks of treatment, all doctors are expected to do so; only then, they hold, can the patient make an intelligent decision as to whether he will subject himself to treatment. This is the doctrine of informed consent. It has many ramifications of importance for the cosmetic surgeon and for all other physicians, for that matter. One is that it does not absolve the physician from negligence and, in fact, permits awards for damages to patients for injuries not caused by negligent medical treatment.

There are several types of consent:

1. Express consent, which may be oral or written
2. Implied consent, which may be implied by action or in an emergency; two factors must be present to constitute an emergency; there must be an immediate danger of death or serious bodily injury, and the patient must be unable to give his consent
3. Consent of a parent or guardian, required for a minor
4. Consent of a guardian, required for the mentally incompetent

A patient's consent is considered informed if he is legally and mentally capable of giving it, if he understands English, if the least technical language possible has been used by the physician, and if it is given after he has had an opportunity to ask questions that had been answered in a satisfactory manner. The patient should understand the following:

1. The nature of the condition
2. The nature and purpose of the proposed treatment
3. The possible alternative treatments
4. The risks or consequences of both the proposed and alternative treatments
5. The chances of failure of the proposed and alternative treatments
6. That no guarantee of success is given

A blanket consent form that authorizes a physician to do whatever he thinks best may be worthwhile because it contains no indication that the patient's consent was informed.

It should be evident that the whole matter of informed consent hinges on risk disclosure by the physician and voluntary acceptance of risk by the patient. In addition, it should be apparent that, even though the patient fails to ask about risks before treatment, a surgeon may be held liable for failing to disclose them on the legal theory that the patient would not have consented to the procedure if he had known of the risks.

A surgeon cannot possibly appraise the patient of all the risks he must assume because they infinite in number; he must be informed, however, to the extent that a "reasonable" person may be enabled to make a decision. No infallible guidelines exist for every situation that may be encountered in practice; they may vary according to the circumstances of the case and the accepted standards of practice for such cases.

Three things are certain, however: first, if a procedure is plagued by a well-recognized hazard or risk of failure (as in cosmetic surgery wherein, as we have already noted, the measure of success is the patient's, not the physician's, satisfaction), disclosure is mandatory; second, the less the immediate need for a proposed procedure, the greater should be the disclosure of risks; and third, physicians should not be evasive or withhold information when direct questions are asked by the patient.

Some proceed on the theory that a physician is under no legal obligation to explain to the average patient what a reasonably informed person should already know; in fact, some courts have confirmed this by holding that patients can be expected to know that there are some risks in any operations or in any anesthetic procedure. However, this would seem to be a very risky assumption and is not recommended.

Consent should also be secured for the administration of anesthetics, for the taking and possible publication of photographs, for having medical visitors in the operating room during surgery, for additional procedures that form a reasonable and customary part or extension of the treatment, for measures that are reasonably necessary to remedy or repair unforseen findings or consequences of the treatment consented to, and for the use of tissue grafts or implants. The surgeon should understand that consent does not extend to procedures that are not part of the treatment consented to.

It is generally conceded wise to have every patient who is to undergo surgery sign a formal consent form and have this signature witnessed by a third person, usually an office assistant. Some doctors, even in the face of our legal climate, are still reluctant to do this, but we submit that it is much less disquieting than having to defend one's self later in court against charges of battery. Actually, such a form is little more than a formal acknowledgment of the patient-education process, and it is generally agreed that well-informed patients make the best patients in the long run.

A consent form should be tailored to an individual's practice and written in words that patients can reasonably be expected to understand. All blanks in the form should be filled in by the physician personally. Finally, the form should be read to or by the patient in a quiet environment, and he should be given an opportunity to ask further questions before his signature is affixed.

Consent forms cannot protect one against every eventuality, but they do indicate to the courts that an earnest attempt was made to prepare the patient in accordance with legal requirements. Since they are not static things, they should be changed from time to time to reflect new developments in the field. The form we are currently using is displayed in Figure 1.

In the final analysis, informed consent depends on the surgeon's ability to communicate with and educate his patients, and his taking the time to do so. Although some may feel this is unnecessarily burdensome, it pays big dividends because, if he knows of a danger and voluntarily exposes himself to it, a patient is deemed to have assumed the risk and is precluded from recovery for any injury received. The interpretations and application of the doctrine of informed consent varies from jurisdiction to jurisdiction, and it is incumbent on the physician to find out what they are in his locale.

NEGLIGENCE

A physician's treatment must conform to reasonable standards; if it does not, and a patient can prove that an injury occurred as a result of it, the physician is liable for negligence. Courts consider four elements necessary for negligence to occur:

1. The person must be accepted as a patient, that is, a contract must be made; a physician is not legally bound to accept anyone as a patient.
2. The physician's treatment did not meet approved standards of care; this is usually established by the testimony of another physician.
3. Improper treatment must result in damage that could reasonably have been forseen; the issue of what is reasonably foreseeable is usually resolved by the jury.
4. A causal connection exists between the breach of care and the damage to the patient.

Standards of care vary according to the circumstances surrounding a particular case. Courts depend on the testimony of other doctors or so-called expert witnesses to determine if recognized and accepted treatments were used and if they met the standard of care. The standards for a specialist, for example, a cosmetic facial surgeon, are considered to be the same wherever they practice. Such standards change when medicine advances, and physicians are expected to keep reasonably abreast of the changes.

Another legal doctrine has evolved in cases in which negligence is at issue, namely, res ipsa loquitur ("the thing speaks for itself"); it holds that the very occurrence of injury in some cases implies that someone, either the defendant physician or someone responsible to him, was careless or negligent. The implication is that the cause of injury was exclusively under the physician's control and that the plaintiff did not contribute to his own injury. Attorneys often claim they invoke this doctrine because of their inability to secure the services of expert witnesses; they claim there is a so-called conspiracy of silence among physicians. If applicability of the doctrine is approved by the judge, the burden of proof is transferred from the patient-plaintiff to the defendant-physician; juries are then instructed that the physician was careless or negligent. The danger is that some courts apply it in cases in which there are unfavorable results, even if there is no negligence.

In addition to carelessness or negligence, physicians may be judged guilty of malpractice on other counts: failure to give adequate instructions for the patient's care after operation, failure to consult, if indicated, concealment, inadequate attention to the case, and abandonment.

A physician may also be held liable for the negligent acts of other people who help him in treating the patient, including his office nurses and assistants, hospital personnel, partners, or, for that matter, anyone whom he asks or invites to assist him whether or not these people are qualified. His liability exists so long as they are under his supervision and control, which they are presumed to be if he was present at the time the negligent act occurred or knew of it and could have prevented it.

Another area in which infractions may occur relates to the patient's right to privacy. Everyone is presumed to have the right to privacy, and the medical contract is considered a private transaction. Neither the physician nor any of his assistants may breach this right of the patient by revealing the existence of any aspect of the physician-patient relationship without the specific written consent of the patient; otherwise, they may be considered guilty of invasion of privacy. This includes using photographs of the patient in any context or permitting colleagues to witness the patient's operation without consent.

Finally, physicians may even be sued for libel (written defamation) or slander (oral defamation) in the course of practice because they make derogatory and malicious statements about patients or colleagues. Defamation violates an individual's right to enjoy a good reputation; this right continues and is available to the individual only so long as, by his conduct, he is entitled to a good reputation. Libel is defamation accomplished by printing or writing; it is considered more serious than slander because it keeps defamation alive for others to see or read, that is, its effect is continuing.

For defamation to be actionable, two requirements must be met: (1) the disparagement must be communicated or published; and (2) there must be malicious intent to harm. Communication is necessary because a person's reputation is based on his standing in the community; malicious intent is necessary to show deliberate purpose on the part of the defamer to cause damage to reputation; in this connection, if the statement he makes is false, malice is automatically presumed.

Any discreditable statememt made about the reputation or character of another that implies unfitness for office or profession is defamation per se; legally, such statements have the effect of cre-

INFORMED CONSENT FOR COSMETIC SURGERY

NAME: _____ DATE _____

1. I hereby request and authorize Dr. Anderson, aided by any assistants he may require, to perform in the presence of qualified medical personnel

_____

_____

upon _____ on or about the _____ day of _____ _____

19_____.

In general terms, the nature and purpose of the operation(s) is:

_____

_____

2. I have read the parts of the booklet entitled COSMETIC SURGERY pertinent to the proposed surgery, and I understand them. Furthermore, Dr. Anderson has fully explained in terms clear to me the effect and nature of the operation(s) to be performed, the forseeable risks involved, alternative methods of treatment as well as what I can expect to experience if recovery is uneventful. Lastly, I acknowledge that I have been given an opportunity to ask any questions I desire regarding the matters covered in the preceeding two sentences and that these questions have been answered to my satisfaction.

3. The risks I was specifically advised of included: temporary swelling and discoloration about the face; the possibility of postoperative bleeding or infection; the development of allergic reactions to medications used during the course of treatment; dissatisfaction with the results of the operation; and the fact that the healing takes longer in some people than in others. In accordance with Louisiana law, I was reminded that in any operation deaths have been known to occur from anesthesia, that the functions of such organs as the brain, eyes, ears, lungs, intestines, kidneys, etc., have been adversely affected, and paralysis of limbs or other parts of the body can occur, and that scars sometimes widen or become otherwise enlarged. Finally, I was told that numberless other complications are possible.

4. I also authorize the operating surgeon to perform any other procedures which he may deem necessary or desirable in attempting to achieve the object of the operation(s) or the elimination of any unhealthy or unforseen condition that he may encounter during the operation(s).

5. I consent to the administration of anesthetics to be applied by or under the direction of Dr. Anderson and to the use of such anesthetics and medications as he may deem advisable in my case.

6. I have been advised that the object of the operation I have requested is improvement in appearance, not perfection, that there is the possibility that imperfections might ensue, and that the result might not live up to my expectations or the goals that have been established. In this connection, I know that the practice of medicine and surgery is not an exact science and that, therefore, reputable physicians cannot guarantee results. I acknowledge that no guarantee or assurance has been made by anyone regarding the operation(s) which I have herein requested and authorized.

7. I have been advised that part of this surgery is — may be — performed through external incisions in the skin which will leave permanent scars whose extent and location have been described to me. I have been advised that scars take upwards of one year to mature, and the changes that normally occur in their appearance during the healing period have been described to me. The location of scars have been indicated to me by one of the doctors at the bottom of this form.

8. I have been told that a medical grade plastic implant will be used in the above-mentioned operation and have been advised of the risks as well as alternative methods of treatment.

9. I have been informed that the above operation may require transplantation of
from other areas of my body or from other persons.

10. I hereby give permission to Dr. Anderson or any assistant he may designate to take photographs for diagnostic purposes and to enhance the medical record. I agree that these photographs will remain their property. I further authorize them to use such photographs for teaching purposes or to illustrate scientific papers, books, or lectures if, in their judgement medical research, education or science will be benefitted by their use; it is specifically understood that in any such publication or use I shall not be identified by name.

11. I understand that if Dr. Anderson judges at any time that my surgery should be postponed or cancelled for any reasons, they may do so.

12. I agree to follow the instructions given to me by Dr. Anderson to the best of my ability before, during and after the above named surgical procedure.

13. I hereby state that the information furnished Dr. Anderson during my diagnostic evaluation is correct.

(Date): _____ / _____ / _____   (Signed): _____
                                              (Patient or person authorized to
                                              give consent for the patient)

                                     (Signed): _____
                                              (Patient if minor)

(Witness): _____
           (not a member of the family)

    I certify that all blanks in the above form were filled in prior to the above signatures and I explained them to the patient or his representative before requesting the patient or his representative to sign the form

                                     _____
                                              (signature of physician)

LOCATION OF INCISIONS

(NOTE: The patient, or his authorized representative, should initial the drawings where incisions have been indicated.)

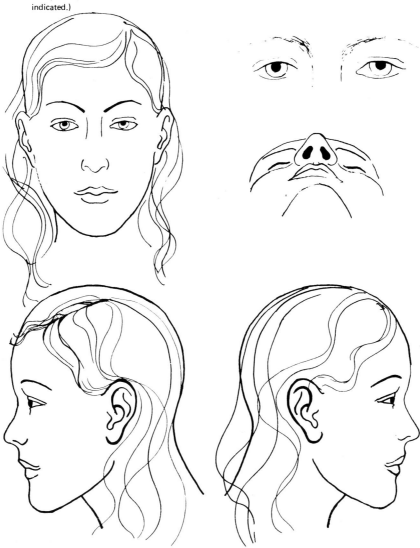

Figure 1. Informed consent form. Any external incisions to be made are indicated on diagrams of face and initialed by the patient before surgery.

ating an immediate damaging opinion in the minds of those who hear or read them. In an action for defamation per se, damages need not be proved — they are inferred from the gravity of the charge. On the other hand, any statement that ridicules or defames another person or group or holds them up to public contempt is libel per se.

Protection against these hazards is often not covered in professional liability policies; separate coverage must be purchased. Every cosmetic surgeon encounters patients who are, to put it mildly, "peculiar" and sees poor results of colleagues for whom he has antipathy. Careless talk or succumbing to the temptation to vent one's spleen can prove unwise in such instances.

MALPRACTICE SELF-PROTECTION AND AVOIDANCE

Patients make claims against physicians for several reasons:

1. They feel that an injury, real or imagined, has occurred during the course of their treatment or that the physician has done something without their knowledge or consent.
2. They are dissatisfied with the results obtained; this may be initiated or abetted by the reactions of others, such as physicians, nurses, family, friends, or attorneys.
3. There has been a breakdown in interpersonal relations that causes them to become angry and want to "punish" the physician.
4. They may see litigation as a way to obtain "easy" money.

There is no secret formula that gives immunity to malpractice claims, nor is there any reliable way to identify the "claims-prone" patient. That we live in a litiginous society is a fact that cosmetic surgeons must face and accept if they want to continue pursuing their calling.

One way of coping with the situation is to practice "defensive medicine." This consists of knowing the hazards that exist, avoiding them in advance to the greatest extent possible, being alert to detect the earliest signs that danger is imminent during tretment, and being ready to take appropriate remedial action without hesitation as soon as the hazard is detected. The practice of good medicine and good interpersonal relations is mandatory; that is about all one can do. Even so,

every cosmetic surgeon can expect to be sued eventually if he practices long enough or if his practice volume is large enough.

Relative to this, doctors should view lawyers realistically.

A malpractice case is an emotional upheaval for a doctor, but it is little more than a chance to earn a fee to an attorney. Unless he is unsophisticated, the lawyer will weigh his expenses and the amount of his time that will be involved against the possibility of winning and the size of the recovery. They usually do not accept cases unless the unsatisfactory result is obvious, that is, it does not fall within the range of acceptable results, the monetary recovery potential is substantial, and the case has dramatic possibilities in court. However, some attorneys file suits that seem to have little merit in the hope that a scared and timid doctor will settle out of court, and, thus, they might reap a good fee quickly without having much work to do.

Taking into consideration the difficulties sometimes inherent in patient selection, the complexity of the procedures, the factors outside the surgeon's control (such as the effect of healing), and the fact that patients may expect too much, it is really amazing that cosmetic surgeons are not sued more often than they are; it speaks well for their awareness and attention to the problem.

The following are some of the malpractice self-protective measures that should be considered.

In general:

1. Have adequate professional liability insurance coverage consistent with current awards.
2. Keep abreast of latest medical advances to the best of one's ability.
3. Practice defensive medicine.
4. Avoid loose talk about patients and colleagues.
5. Make a studied attempt to practice good interpersonal relations; try to establish good rapport with the patient from the very beginning, since it has often been said that most malpractice actions result from some breakdown of interpersonal relations; do not be rude, ignore patients, or treat them as numbers.

Before surgery, the following should be considered:

1. Select patients carefully from both psychologic and physical standpoints.

2. Do not accept for operation patients with whom good rapport cannot be established, patients who do not emanate "good vibes."
3. Obtain and check all indicated laboratory reports and consultations.
4. Be sure the patient is legally competent to contract for surgery.
5. Do not "oversell" procedures, be unnecessarily enthusiastic, or give an expressed or implied warranty.
6. Satisfy the requirements of the doctrine of informed consent by educating patients personally and with printed material; prepare them for what to expect; answer all questions truthfully, directly, and without evasion.
7. Educate the patient and those who will be caring for the patient about the details of postoperative care.
8. Discuss the surgical fee in advance, what it covers, and when payment is due; have the patient sign an acknowledgement of this; hostility over a bill is often a patient's way of expressing displeasure.
9. Take preoperative photographs.
10. Have the patient sign a consent form tailored to your practice; do not depend on the hospital consent form; keep all signed consent forms in a safe place, not in the patient's file.
11. Record all pertinent material in the patient's chart; it is almost impossible to prove that you did something or looked for something unless it is recorded; it has been said that the best defense is a written defense — anything that is not in writing is hearsay.

During hospitalization and surgery, the following should be done:

1. Keep good records that include material relevant to the patient's condition and that fairly portrays a treatment that meets the standard of practice; check patient's charts daily.
2. See that all necessary operating room equipment is available and in good working order and that you know how to use it.
3. Monitor the vital signs of all patients during surgery, even if the operation is done under local anesthesia.
4. Attempt only those procedures within your capability; avoid new procedures with unknown risks or experimental operations.
5. Do nothing the hospital permit does not specify.
6. Monitor the activities of assistants, nurse anesthetists, and anesthesiologists.

After discharge from the hospital, do the following:

1. Keep good records.
2. See the patient as often as the practice of good medicine dictates; note at the end of each visit when the patient is to return.
3. Have office assistants note broken appointments on the patient's chart.
4. Closely supervise the activities of office assistants who take part in postoperative care.
5. Give adequate emotional support.
6. Advise patients of any untoward developments, and care for them without fanfare.
7. Be available; notify patients of any necessary unavailability and the doctor who is covering during your absence.
8. Never discharge a patient who complains of pain, swelling, or a "funny feeling"; discharge means treatment is terminated, that nothing more can be done.
9. Keep copies of all correspondence, including insurance forms.
10. If dissatisfaction arises, avoid becoming hostile; hear the patient out and give adequate emotional support and respect; then, give him facts, answers, and understanding; tell him what can be done and what cannot be done; never take hope away; record all patient grievances.
11. If it appears that a malpractice action is imminent, obtain legal advice immediately; make no oral or written statements to the patient, his family, or his attorneys until such legal advice is secured. Do not make changes in the patient's records; one of the most disastrous things that can happen to a doctor in court is for the plaintiff's attorney to bring out the fact that the records have been changed and argue to the jury that they would not have been changed if the doctor did not feel he was negligent.

Two final points concern relations with attorneys. First, plaintiff attorneys nowadays are not only looking at reports to help them in the suit against the party that injured his client initially, they are also looking at them for possible malpractice charges against the doctor who rendered secondary treatment. Secondly, physicians should be very cautious in conferences with attorneys representing their patients after accidents. Whereas on the surface they may appear to want the conference to get information about the patient to file suit against the person who has caused an accident, here again, the attorneys will be looking for elements of malpractice. As a matter of fact, attorneys nationally have been urged through their literature to have conferences with doctors for this very purpose.

4   Patient Selection: Psychologic and Physical Considerations

At some time during their careers, most rhinoplasty surgeons have remarked, "In retrospect, I guess I shouldn't have operated on that patient." Perhaps they were not satisfied with the result, or, maybe, it was the patient who was displeased. In either case, it underscores the importance of careful patient selection for surgery.

Many experienced surgeons rate the selection process more difficult than the surgery itself. On the other hand, young surgeons, perhaps because of their inexperience or because of their natural eagerness to operate, are often more unwary in the choice of patients. This is unfortunate because careful selection is in the best interest of both the doctor and the patient; it may prevent much disquiet and unpleasantness later on in the relationship.

Not every person seeking cosmetic surgery is a good candidate. Certain patients are psychologically unfit, no matter how much they want it and no matter how amenable their deformities are to correction; others should not be operated on because of physical factors. It should be apparent, then, that it is just as important for the surgeon to know when not to operate as when to operate.

Finally, the possibility exists that appearance may not be the only reason for the patient's discontent. He may undergo surgery, obtain results that are generally conceded to be successful and still not achieve the happiness he seeks. Furthermore, his evaluation of the result is highly subjective and uncertain, may be strongly affected by the attitude of others, and depends largely on self-acceptance. Cosmetic surgery, then, has more psychologic overtones than other types of surgery, and the cosmetic surgeon must be prepared to deal with the psychologic as well as the physical condition of patients.

PSYCHOLOGIC CONSIDERATIONS

Acceptable candidates for rhinoplasty should have good motivations, realistic expectations, and sufficient ego strength to undergo the procedure, the rigors of the postoperative period, the risk of complications, and the possibility that the outcome may not be satisfying to them.

In general, it might be said that if a patient indicates that correction of a specific deformity will help him feel better about his appearance and, so, enable him to be more at ease psychologically and function better socially, his motivation is probably acceptable. Actually, such an individual is seeking to rid himself of a belief on which he has been expending excessive psychic energy so that he might spend it more effectively elsewhere; incidentally, the amount of psychic emphasis may not be proportional to the size of the deformity.

On the other hand, if his motivation is not egocentric, that is, if he expects the operation to alter the attitudes or responses of others toward him so that he will be better liked, more successful, or more secure, he will be a poor candidate for surgery. This is also true if he is seeking correction to please someone else or because of a rivalry for another's attention, approval, or affection.

The history should be taken unhurriedly. A frank appraisal of the patient is made during its unfolding in an attempt to discover whether he/she is depressed, if his/her behavior is disorganized or inappropriate, or if a female seems seductive or manipulative.

The following questions should always be asked directly, and the surgeon should guard against being taken in by oversimplification or incompleteness since this may mask deeper motivations. Therefore the patient should be asked to elaborate further if the collection of more information seems indicated.

What type of surgery are you considering?

The surgeon must not fall into the trap of assuming he knows what the patient wants. Likewise, what the patient wants and what the surgeon thinks he needs may be quite different; nevertheless, unless the surgeon's suggestions are solicited, they should not be offered to the patient until the relationship progresses further.

What specific features do you want corrected?

If the patient's attitude is realistic and coincides with what is possible technically, the surgery should produce a satisfied patient. Therefore straightforward answers are the best; vagueness indicates that there may be another reason for the patient's discontent and that he may be erroneously ascribing it to his deformity.

How long have you been thinking about having surgery?

It is better if a person's decision to have surgery is well thought out, not a spur of the moment thing. Rashness is one characteristic of hypomania or manic-depressive states. Such patients may impulsively rush out for surgery while doing a thousand other things and, then, either go into a deep depression or regret the surgery later.

What caused you to begin thinking about it?

The answer given to this question will reveal whether or not the patient is taking the matter lightly; the longer he has been considering the possibility of surgery, the better. Sometimes, the nidus was planted by teasing during childhood, or, perhaps, it began when the patient saw his profile in a photo or a mirror. Casual remarks by hairdressers often initiate the process.

Why do you want the operation at this time?

Not being able to afford surgery previously or the inability to take time off from work or school are good reasons; so is the fact that deterioration had not progressed far enough until recent date. Examples of invalid reasons would include seeking operation to relieve depression caused by the death of a mate, the break-up of a love affair, or some similar crisis.

Why do you want the operation?

Good motivations might include: improve appearance, eliminate self-consciousness and teasing, permit more effective use of cosmetics and hair styles, improve one's chances in the job market, eliminate an unpleasant family characteristic, or look better for one's age. To please or impress others, to relieve depressed feelings, or to compensate for patent inferiority would be unacceptable reasons.

What other cosmetic operations have you had? Were you satisfied with the results?

These questions can help uncover surgical masochists, appearance neurotics, and those with such widespread discontent and such poor self-images that even multiple surgeries are not likely to be helpful. The patient's reaction to the results of previous cosmetic surgery is important information for the surgeon to assimilate in deciding whether or not to accept him for the operation he seeks. Our impression has been that people who have had multiple operations seem less happy, feel less self-confident, and have worse self-images than those who had only one or even those who had never yet been operated on.

What is the attitude of your family and friends to the proposed operation?

If those persons who are close to the patient approve the operation, they usually provide helpful support when the patient is coping with the morbidity that everyone must endure; disapproving feedback during the postoperative period, on the other hand, can be very destructive and can sorely tax the physician-patient relationship. Tacit approval of mates and other close relatives is almost a necessity.

A number of other facts of psychologic importance should be kept in mind. Certainly, having surgery should be the patient's own idea; it should not be sought to please someone else because that person may find yet other things to become dissatisfied with once the deformity is corrected. Also, since the patient failed to gain the acceptance and love he wanted or needed, he may become depressed or may seek to blame someone, perhaps the surgeon.

A neurosis does not contraindicate surgery, for most of us are neurotic to some extent. The simple neurotic person is recognized by his worry, his anxiousness, and his somatic symptoms. Such an individual is usually aware of his stress, and his symptoms diminish when he discusses his problems. He gets better (unlike the hysterical patient, for example) as a result of the surgeon's attention, respect, and reassurance, so he usually makes a good patient, although supportive counseling may be indicated in some cases before and after the operation.

Depression is the most common emotional disturbance in the general population; varying degrees are encountered by the cosmetic surgeon, and they may have serious implications for him. He is rarely or never consulted by the psychotically depressed individual who has lost all hope and self-esteem and really does not care about his appearance.

On the other hand, the neurotically depressed are frequently encountered. Such people are sad and hope that the cosmetic surgeon can help them regain happiness, erase their pessimism, improve their self-esteem, and make them lovable again. Frequently, there is a large element of inexpressable anger and guilt associated with the condition. Surgery should be postponed until the depression is treated because the attendant physical and emotional stress may increase the patient's depression.

Two recommendations are worth considering. Psychiatric clearance should be sought for everyone who has previously attempted suicide or who has been treated for depression in the past with drugs, shock treatment, or psychotherapy. Those depressed individuals who are secretly hoping to die from the procedure should, of course, be refused operation; such a desire may surface after the patient is told he is depressed and a psychiatric consultation is required; incidentally, depressed patients are usually surprisingly amenable to psychiatric consultation.

A large number of hysterically neurotic patients consult cosmetic surgeons. They usually are warm and interesting people, although immature. They tend to be artistically inclined, to exaggerate physical symptoms, and their problems seem to be exaggerated with attention. They look to the surgeon to take total responsibility and, even, to perform miracles ("I'll leave it entirely up to you doctor. Do what you think best."). Such individuals usually do not respond well to counseling because of their immaturity.

As is well known, the obsessively compulsive and neurotic patient exhibits phobic behavior and rigid, ritualistic thought and actions. He fabricates a web of rationalization and tends to communicate lengthily ad nauseam. Discussions with him are best kept simple and factual. If he "buys" the surgeons approach, he usually becomes a good patient; if he does not, his request should be refused.

Fortunately, the number of psychotic patients seeking cosmetic surgery is low, but it is absolutely necessary to ferret out paranoid patients who focus the blame for all disappointments and failures in their lives on some cosmetic defect; if they become dissatisfied, which is almost inevitable, they frequently become defamatory and litiginous and may even resort to violence against the physician. These people, without exception, should be denied surgery.

When the interviewing physician feels as though he is dealing with an enigma and as though he himself is becoming disoriented, he is probably being consulted by a person with a schizoid personality. Their symptoms range from unusual to bizarre and distorted thoughts to peculiar behavior. Such people may benefit from cosmetic surgery, but they pose a surgical risk because they may not have sufficient ego strength to withstand elective surgery without counseling. Incidentally, some surgeons feel that there is a high incidence of schizoid tendencies in men who seek rhinoplasty.

Patients with personality disorders (inadequate personality, psychopathically deviant personality, sociopathic personality) tend to become dissatisfied, litiginous, and critical and they may resort to violence. Initially, they may appear intelligent, independent, interesting, and challenging; at the same time, they are subtly seducing the surgeon into satisfying their infantile wishes, or they are manipulating him into feeling all-powerful and then conning him into attempting to perform a personality change. Actually, these people have an emotional deficit, that is, they lack warmth or deep emotional response, and they try to solve their internal problems by external means (for example, cosmetic surgery); the problem they pose to the surgeon is that they tend to act out their problems rather than internalizing them. They have two important characteristics: they are adept at disguising their pathologic condition, and they are expert at tapping the narcissistic and power needs of other unsuspecting persons. In fact, no cosmetic surgeon can supply what these patients lack, so any effort would be doomed to failure.

Finally, many advise steering clear of people who wish correction of minor cosmetic defects. They contend that such a defect is more likely to be symbolic of an emotional conflict that cannot be cured by surgery. Our experience has been that no constant relationship exists between the size of the deformity and the amount of stress it produces. Although it is true that the margin for error is smaller in the correction of a small deformity, and more judgment and finesse is usually required, some of the most mutually pleasing results have been obtained in such cases after good, careful patient preparation.

CAUTION SIGNALS IN THE HISTORY

A "Caution!" signal should begin flashing in the surgeon's mind if he elicits any of the following during an interview:

1. Vagueness about the correction desired.
2. Evidence of rashness in the patient's decision-making process.

3. Poor motivation.
4. Unrealistic expectation. For example the patient expects the rhinoplasty to make her beautiful; he feels that an entire career revolves around the success or failure of the operation; a deep sense of inferiority is attributed to a deformity and the operation is expected to correct this; the patient expects to retrieve a lost lover or marriage partner as a result of the operation.
5. A history of having had multiple cosmetic operations in the past.
6. Dissatisfaction with previous cosmetic operations with disparagement of the surgeons involved and a history of legal action.
7. Active disapproval of the undertaking by those with whom the patient lives.
8. The surgery is being sought to please others.
9. The desire for surgery began with some recent emotional crisis.
10. Evidence that considerable depression may exist, a history of previous treatment of depression with drugs, shock treatment, or psychotherapy, or, finally, suicide has been attempted in the past.
11. A history of prolonged psychiatric counseling or psychoanalysis in the past, or therapy that the patient is presently undergoing.
12. The patient appears to have an infantile narcissistic or manipulative personality.
13. The correction is required for a minor defect or virtually nonexistent defects.
14. The patient exhibits a perfectionistic attitude by attempting to establish detailed specifications and to exact specific assurance.
15. The patient says, "I'll leave it up to you. Do what you want with it."
16. The patient evinces intense urgency for correction of a long-standing deformity.
17. The request for cosmetic surgery is made under the guise of seeking physiologic improvement.
18. The patient is making an attempt to circumvent or bypass the established routine of the surgeon.
19. The patient is excessively secretive or indecisive.
20. Requests for cosmetic rhinoplasty from men. Some surgeons believe there is a high incidence of schizoid tendencies among such patients and that their hopes and expectations are apt to be unrealistic.

As was mentioned previously, almost everyone has some degree of neurosis in certain areas, but these may be realistic responses to external situations and pose no contraindication to surgery. The problem is for the surgeon to determine the magnitude and significance of the aberrations. Psychiatric consultation is indicated if he feels unable to do so.

Davis has pointed out that the goal of psychiatric screening is not meant to eliminate the neurotic patient from having surgery; it is to eliminate only those who are likely to have an unhappy result. Unfortunately, not every psychiatrist understands the issues involved in screening patients for cosmetic surgery; in fact, it is unfair to expect him to do so on the basis of a 45 minute consultation. Therefore the surgeon should select one psychiatrist in his area, familiarize him with the work, and ask that he review some of the pertinent literature, of which there is an abundance in order to improve his insight and, so, the help he can render.

Shulman has formulated the questions the psychiatric consultant should be able to answer for the cosmetic surgeon:

1. Is the patient mentally ill? If so, should the surgery go on anyway? With what precautions?
2. Does the patient have hidden fantasies about the surgery so that it is highly unlikely he will be a satisfied patient? Is it impossible for surgery to really accomplish the patient's objective?
3. Will the surgery lead to decompensation (a breakdown of defenses with resulting psychic problems)?
4. Does this patient have a tendency to be litiginous, accusing, or angry at the surgeon and the hospital?
5. Will the patient change his mind and regret the surgery? Is his motivation too shaky? Is it unrealistic?
6. Can the patient accept less than perfection? Will he be deeply disappointed if the result is a little different from what he expected?

PSYCHIATRIC CONSULTATION — REFUSING OPERATION

One of the most frequent questions asked during instruction courses is, "How do you get a patient to consult a psychiatrist?." The second most common is, "How do you turn a patient down for surgery?". Psychiatric referral requires diplomacy. We usually tell patients that we are unsure whether they could withstand the rigors of the operation, that they may be too "nervous." We fear it might be harmful if they did and would not like to chance the risk. We then tell them that, since we are not experts in evaluating such matters, we would like them to be evaluated by a consultant (a psychiatrist).

The suggestion is usually readily accepted by those who have had previous counseling. It is, also, usually accepted by those who are depressed and those who feel we have a genuine concern for their welfare. A few reject our request, in which case we are probably better off in the long run.

To turn down a patient's request for surgery, we simply say that we do not think we could get a good result for them. A patient would have to be an utter fool to persist in trying to obtain the services of a doctor who felt incapable of obtaining improvement for them, and their persistence would only reinforce the wisdom of the decision.

PHYSICAL CONSIDERATIONS

One of the happiest circumstances about rhinoplastic surgery or any cosmetic surgery, for that matter, is that it is elective. The surgeon is not called on to take calculated risks resulting from the presence of other conditions, serious or not, that the patient might have. Every significant factor can be checked. If anything abnormal is found, operation can be denied or deferred to some later, more favorable time. This presupposes that an adequate history is taken on every patient before operation.

Evidence of infection anywhere in the body, but especially in the head and neck area, should cause postponement of surgery, even if it is not discovered until the patient comes to the operating suite. People who have asthma or any chronic lung or bronchial condition should be carefully considered from the standpoint of the effects of anesthetic agents and postoperative coughing. Anyone with a history of heart disease or high blood pressure should be referred to his family doctor or to a cardiologist for clearance and advice, since epinephrine is usually used in rhinoplasty for hemostatic purposes. A history of any liver disease or dysfunction should be elicited, not only from the standpoint of drug and anesthetic metabolism, but, also, because hepatitis is so prevalent today as a result of the drug subculture.

Direct questions should be asked concerning any history of diabetes, epilepsy, chronic dermatitis, unexplained gain or loss of weight, bleeding tendencies, and drug or anesthetic allergies or idiosyncracies (particularly to drugs the surgeon expects to use before, during, and after the operation). A review should also be made of the drugs the patient frequently uses, whether as a result of physician's prescription or of his own volition. It is well to inquire if there is a history of poor scarring after previous operations or trauma and of past reactions to any type of suture material or adhesive tape. A history of past operations the patient has undergone and their postoperative recovery may be illuminating. Finally, it is wise to determine if the patient is currently dieting because some of the popular high-protein diets interfere with the blood-clotting mechanism and predispose to excessive bruising and bleeding.

The aesthetic improvement possible may be limited by certain features found in the nose itself. Included are: concomitant septal deformities; serious nasal allergy; thick skin and subcutaneous tissues; flaccid cartilages; infantile tip projection; excessive size or width; excessive projection from the face; short columella; webbing of the columella base; nostrils that are too small or too large, particularly if their long axes approach the horizontal; and nostrils that lack sills. Aesthetic improvement is also prejudiced by a history of multiple nasal trauma or previous operations.

USE OF A SELF-ADMINISTERED HISTORY QUESTIONNAIRE

To save time and to ensure thoroughness in the collection of information that might be important in a prospective patient's history, we developed a self-administered history questionnaire (Fig. 2) that has been used thousands of times during the past 10 years. The closed-end questions contained therein were carefully designed so that the average patient would have no trouble answering them; they are supplemented, when indicated, during consultation by conventional open-ended questions.

The questionnaire elicits the following informatin about every patient who consults us for cosmetic surgery: (1) motivations, (2) expectations, (3) prior knowledge about the procedures, (4) habits, (5) present physical condition, (6) past medical history, (7) tolerance for drugs we usually use, (8) a listing of the medications currently being taken, and (9) personality. Finally, as a mediocolegal self-protective device, additional questions have been interwoven among the medical ones to establish that the patient has been told that the object of such surgery is improvement, not perfection, that no guarantees have been given, that risks must be assumed, and that morbidity is to be expected.

The questionnaire is sent to the patient's home when he calls to schedule his initial consultation.

COSMETIC SURGERY EVALUATION INVENTORY

Cosmetic surgery should not be considered lightly simply because it's purpose is to improve appearance rather than to eradicate disease or save lives; like any other surgery, it entails risks. Therefore, anyone contemplating it must be physically healthy and able to cope with it emotionally.

This questionnaire was designed to collect a great deal of information about your physical condition, past medical history, habits, personality, etc., that will enable us to advise you whether or not it would be wise for you to have cosmetic surgery at the present time.

During your consultation we will review the completed form together and explore further any areas which seem to require amplification.

Your answers will remain confidential, as will all other aspects of your association with this office and members of our Staff.

NAME: (print) _____ AGE: _____

HOME ADDRESS: _____ CITY, ZIP: _____

EDUCATION: (highest year of school compelted) _____

OCCUPATION: _____ HOW LONG? _____

Please circle below the type of surgery you are considering:

NOSE	CHIN	LIPS
EYELIDS	FACE	NECK
EARS	FACE PEEL	SCARS

OTHER: _____

1. What specific features do you want corrected?

_____

2. How long have you been thinking about having surgery?

_____

3. What caused you to begin thinking about it?

_____

4. Is having surgery your idea or is it someone else's idea?

_____

5. Why did you wait until now to come in for the correction?

_____

6. Have you read articles in newspapers, magazines or books about cosmetic surgery?   Yes No

7. Do you understand that the object of any cosmetic operation is improvement in appearance, not perfection?   Yes No

8. Has anyone in your family or a friend had cosmetic surgery?   Yes No

   If they did, what was done?

   _____

   Did you discuss the operation with them?   Yes No

9. Do you feel rather embarassed or guilty about having the operation?   Yes No

10. If you have the operation, who do you think will be the happiest with the results?

_____

Check below the reasons why you want the operation:

- ☐ To improve my appearance
- ☐ To eliminate self-consciousness about my appearance
- ☐ Have an inferiority complex about my appearance
- ☐ It makes me look ugly
- ☐ Because people tease me or make derogatory remarks
- ☐ To improve function
- ☐ So I can make up better
- ☐ So I can use different hair styles
- ☐ To help me get or keep a job
- ☐ To help me look better for my age
- ☐ To please or impress others
- ☐ To give me a psychological uplift
- ☐ To make me look more masculine or feminine
- ☐ To please a relative or friend
- ☐ To make me beautiful or handsome
- ☐ To cause other people to react better to me
- ☐ To help achieve certain career goals
- ☐ To help solve personal problems
- ☐ To relieve my depressed feelings
- ☐ To help me solve certain personal problems
- ☐ Because of a family resemblance I dislike
- ☐ I get few compliments about my looks
- ☐ To improve my relations with the opposite sex
- ☐ My looks prevent achievement of certian goals
- ☐ Because of dissatisfaction with previous surgery
- ☐ Because I look dissapated or tired
- ☐ Because I feel young; I want to look younger
- ☐ To help my career
- ☐ To give perfection to my looks

☐ To make other things in my life better   Other reasons _____

_____

_____

11. Do you have any preconceived idea of how you would like your nose, face, etc., to look?   Yes No

If yes, how?

_____

12. Do you realize that every operation is followed by a period of healing before the tissues return to normal and the final result is apparent?   Yes No

13. Are you aware that the possibility exists that the results of the operation might not fully meet your expectations?   Yes No

14. List below any previous cosmetic operations you have had:

_____

_____

Were you satisfied with the results?   Yes No

If not, why not?

_____

_____

15. Are you presently single, married, separated, divorced, or widowed?

_____

How may times have you been married?

_____

How may children do you have?

_____

16. Do you live alone or with someone else (family, friends)?

_____

Have you spoken to your family or friends of your desire for surgery?   Yes No

If not, do you mind if they know?   Yes No

If you have, what is their attitude?

_____

_____

_____

_____

_____

17. Do you:

drink more than 6 cups of coffee or tea daily?   Yes No

smoke more than a pack of cigarettes a day?   Yes No

take more than 2 alcoholic drinks every day?   Yes No

use pot, uppers, downers regularly?   Yes No

use LSD or heroin?   Yes No

have any hobbies?   Yes No

spend much time socializing with friends, family, etc.   Yes No

Medical Evaluation

18. How is your general health?

_____

19. Are you under the care of a doctor for anything at the present time?   Yes No

If not, should you be but have been putting off consulting one?   Yes No

20. When was your last physical examination?

_____

Was everything O.K.?   Yes No

21. Do you seem to be ill more frequently than other people you know?   Yes No

22. Are you having any trouble with your teeth or gums?   Yes No

23. Do you wear partial or complete dentures?   Yes No

24. Do you suffer with recurring fever blisters   Yes No

25. Do you wear eyeglasses or contacts or feel you need them?   Yes No

26. Do you experience recurring eye pain?   Yes No

27. Have you ever had loss of vision?   Yes No

28. Do you suffer with blurring or misty vision?   Yes No

29. Do you see rainbow rings around lights?   Yes No

30. Are you being treated for glaucoma?   Yes No

31. Do you suffer with dryness of the eyes?   Yes No

32. Do you have any other eye complaints?   Yes No

33. Have you ever broken your nose?   Yes No

34. Do you have any chronic nose or sinus complaints?   Yes No

35. Do you have frequent headaches?   Yes No

36. Do you have any chronic ear complaints?   Yes   No

37. Have you ever had facial paralysis?   Yes   No

38. Have you ever had an operation on your face?   Yes   No

39. Do you have asthma or any chronic lung or bron-chian condition?   Yes   No

40. Do you experience recurrent chest pains?   Yes   No

41. Have you ever been told you have any trouble with your heart?   Yes   No

42. Do you have any abdominal problems (stomach, intestinal, gall bladder, liver, hernia, etc.)?   Yes   No

43. Any trouble with your kidneys, bladder, or re-productive system?   Yes   No

44. Any bone, joint or muscular trouble?   Yes   No

45. Do you have any chronic skin condition?   Yes   No

46. Do you have any of the following: diabetes, epi-lepsy, or high blood pressure?   Yes   No

47. Have you ever had a nervous breakdown?   Yes   No

48. Have you ever been under the care of a psychia-trist or psychologist?   Yes   No

49. Has there been any recent emotional crisis in you life?   Yes   No

50. Have you ever been dissatisfied with the treatment you received from a doctor or dentist?   Yes   No

51. Have you had any marked loss or gain of weight lately?   Yes   No

52. Are you on a special diet at the present time?   Yes   No

53. Do you bruise easier than most other people?   Yes   No

54. Do bruises seem to take longer to clear up for you than for most people you know?   Yes   No

55. Do your cuts bleed longer than those other people have?   Yes   No

56. Have you ever had any bleeding episode that re-quired the attention of a doctor?   Yes   No

57. Have you ever had excessive bleeding more than once during your life?   Yes   No

58. Have you ever had hemmorrhage following minor surgery?   Yes   No

59. Have you suffered with recurrent nose bleeds?   Yes   No

60. (FOR WOMEN) Do your periods usually last longer than 4 or 5 days?   Yes   No

61. Have you ever had any of the following operations:

Appendectomy? . . . . .Yes   No
Breast surgery? . . . . .Yes   No
Caesarian section? .Yes   No
Deliveries? . . . . .Yes   No
D & C . . . . .Yes   No
Ear Surgery . . . . .Yes   No
Extraction of teeth? . . . . .Yes   No
Eye surgery? . . . . .Yes   No
Heart surgery? . . . . .Yes   No
Hemorrhoidectomy? . . . . .Yes   No
Hernia repair? . . . . .Yes   No
Hysterectomy? . . . . .Yes   No
Kidney surgery? . . . . .Yes   No
Lung surgery? . . . . .Yes   No
Nose surgery? . . . . .Yes   No
Skin surgery? . . . . .Yes   No
Thyroid surgery? . . . . .Yes   No
Tonsils and adenoids? . . . . .Yes   No
Tumor surgery? . . . . .Yes   No
Others? _____

62. If you have been operated on previously, did you have any unusual bleeding or poor scarring following them or following any injury or fol-lowing vaccination?   Yes   No

63. Did you have a normal recovery following pre-vious surgery?   Yes   No

64. Do you understand that anyone undergoing any operation, even a cosmetic one, must assume certain risks?   Yes   No

65. Do you realize that the results of surgery might not live up to your expectations?   Yes   No

66. As far as you know, have you ever had an aller-gic reaction to any of the following drugs or materials-

Adhesive tape? . . . . .Yes   No
Adrenalin ? . . . . .Yes   No
Antibiotics? . . . . .Yes   No
Antihistamines? . . . . .Yes   No
Atropine? . . . . .Yes   No
Codeine? . . . . .Yes   No
Compazine? . . . . .Yes   No
Cortisone? . . . . .Yes   No
Darvon? . . . . .Yes   No
Demerol? . . . . .Yes   No
Dilaudid? . . . . .Yes   No
Empirin? . . . . .Yes   No
Iodine preparations? . . . . .Yes   No
Local anesthetics (Novocaine, Xylocaine, Cocaine, etc.)? . . . . .Yes   No
Morphine? . . . . .Yes   No
Nembutal? . . . . .Yes   No
Neomycin? . . . . .Yes   No
Seconal? . . . . .Yes   No
Scopolamine (twilight sleep)? . . . . .Yes   No
Suture material? . . . . .Yes   No
Valium? . . . . .Yes   No
Vistaril? . . . . .Yes   No
Others? _____

67. Are you taking any of the following frequently or regularly?:

Allergy shots?......................Yes No
Antibiotics?........................Yes No
Antidepressants?....................Yes No
Antihistamines? ....Yes No
Arthritis medicine? ....Yes No
Aspirin?...........................Yes No
Barbiturates (sleeping pills)? ....Yes No
Birth control pills?..................Yes No
Blood thinners (anticoagulants)? ....Yes No
Blood vessel dilators?.................Yes No
Butazolidin? ....Yes No
Cortisone? ....Yes No
Diabetes medicine? ....Yes No
Diet pills? ....Yes No
Diuretics (fluid pills)?.................Yes No
Epilepsy medicine? ....Yes No
Eye medicine? ....Yes No
Headache remedies?..................Yes No
Heart medicine? ....Yes No
High blood pressure medicine?..........Yes No
Hormones?.........................Yes No
Iron?.............................Yes No
Laxatives? ....Yes No
Mood elevating medicine?..............Yes No
Nose drops? ....Yes No
Pain relievers?......................Yes No
Sleeping pills?......................Yes No
Stomach medicine? ....Yes No
Thyroid?..........................Yes No
Tranquilizers (Librium, Valium, Equanil,
  etc.)?..........................Yes No
Vitamins? ....Yes No
Others:_____

_____

_____

68. Do you react normally to sedation?   Yes No

69. Do some sedative drugs have the opposite   Yes No
effect on you, that is, seem to excite you?

70. Is there a history of any of the following conditions in your family:

Alcoholism?.......................Yes No
Allergies?.........................Yes No
Anesthetic reactions?.................Yes No
Bleeding tendencies? ....Yes No
Cancer?...........................Yes No
Congenital defects? ....Yes No
Eccentricities? ....Yes No
Epilepsy?..........................Yes No
Family estrangements?................Yes No
Heart attacks?......................Yes No
High blood pressure? ....Yes No
Nervous breakdowns?.................Yes No
Stomach trouble? ....Yes No
Strokes? ....Yes No
Suicides?..........................Yes No

71. Are there any reasons you should not have an
an operation at the present time?   Yes No

List below any facts of a medical or other nature which you feel you should make known before you undergo any type of surgery:

_____

_____

_____

_____

_____

_____

_____

72. Have you read the booklet we sent to you (COSMETIC
FACIAL SURGERY)?   Yes No

DATE THIS FORM COMPLETED_____   SIGNATURE:_____

List below any questions you would like to have specifically answered during your consultation:

PERSONALITY INVENTORY

Do you find that you are unhappy, miserable or blue more often than you are happy? □Yes □No

Does life often seem burdensome to you? □Yes □No

Do you often wake up during the night or in early morning and worry? □Yes □No

Do others seem happier than you are? □Yes □No

Are you pessimistic about the future? □Yes □No

Have you been finding it more difficult to concentrate lately? □Yes □No

Do you often feel useless and unable to cope? □Yes □No

Are you hard on yourself, remorseful, and prone to feel guilty? □Yes □No

Do others seem not to be as concerned with the inevitability and grim realities of life as you are? □Yes □No

Do you often have fatigue and other physical symptoms that are difficult to diagnose and relieve? □Yes □No

Do you often feel sad? □Yes □No

Are your outside interests and satisfying relationships with others gradually declining? □Yes □No

Do you often feel alone and sad at parties and other social gatherings? □Yes □No

———

Do you have a tendency to let your imagination "run wild"? □Yes □No

Do you consider yourself a person attuned to the dramatic aspects of life? □Yes □No

Do you consider yourself an artistic or aesthetic person? □Yes □No

(For Women) Are you considered flirtatious, coquettish, seductive — in a word, a sensual type woman? □Yes □No

When someone disagrees with you or disappoints you, is your reaction frequently one of depression or anger? □Yes □No

Is the approval of others very important to you? □Yes □No

Do you require a great deal of affection from others? □Yes □No

Have people complained that you are unpredictable? □Yes □No

Have people said that you are an "exciting" person? □Yes □No

Do you spend a lot of time on your appearance? □Yes □No

Do you find yourself stirring things up so that you become the center of attention or the "life-of-the-party" type? □Yes □No

Are you easily swayed by the suggestions of others? □Yes □No

Are you a very stubborn person? □Yes □No

In your inner life, do you frequently feel insecure and that someone should look after you? □Yes □No

Under stress, does life seem more than you can cope with, and do you frequently develop alarming symptoms at this time? □Yes □No

———

Do you frequently find that certain unwanted words or thoughts persist in running through your mind? □Yes □No

Do you often feel compelled to follow a definite ritual in doing certain things even though you sometimes consider this unreasonable or a waste of time? □Yes □No

Do you prefer to do things yourself rather than delegating them to others? □Yes □No

Do you feel impelled to atone for errors and then find yourself doing the same thing again? □Yes □No

Are you frequently plagued by doubts and uncertainties (examples: did you lock the door before leaving home? did you turn off the lights? did you forget your keys or eyeglasses? etc.) □Yes □No

Do you pride yourself in being:

punctual? □Yes □No

conscientious? □Yes □No

self-critical? □Yes □No

tidy? □Yes □No

orderly? □Yes □No

Are you reserved in social situations and often seem to miss out on the fun? □Yes □No

Do you tend to deny your emotional needs? □Yes □No

Do you consider yourself a proud, strong, independent and reserved type rather than a dependent, warm, and affectionate person? □Yes □No

Do you tend to "bury yourself" in certain activities (for example: your work, club activities, hobbies, religion, etc.) □Yes □No

Do you frequently become impatient with and have to control hostile impulses against "the System", those in authority (parents, teachers, bosses, for example), etc.? □Yes □No

Are you moralistic and often preoccupied with principle? □Yes □No

Do you frequently mistrust others and become suspicious of their intentions? ☐ Yes ☐ No

Do you often feel misunderstood, mistreated or taken advantage of by others? ☐ Yes ☐ No

Do people often complain that you seem to go through life with a chip on your shoulder? ☐ Yes ☐ No

Are you considered opinionated and stubborn? ☐ Yes ☐ No

Do you feel that people often block your free and easy responses by trying to control or influence you? ☐ Yes ☐ No

Down deep, do you consider yourself to be endowed with superior, unique, or unrecognized abilities? ☐ Yes ☐ No

Do you find yourself being envious or jealous of the pleasures and successes of others? ☐ Yes ☐ No

Do you hold grudges? ☐ Yes ☐ No

Are you a "stickler" for going by the rules? ☐ Yes ☐ No

Are you hypersensitive to the opinions of others? ☐ Yes ☐ No

———————

Would you rather be alone than with people most of the time? ☐ Yes ☐ No

Were you considered a quiet, shy, obedient and sensitive child? ☐ Yes ☐ No

Do other people tend to take advantage of you or mistrust you? ☐ Yes ☐ No

Are you an unusually sensitive person easily hurt by others? ☐ Yes ☐ No

Does your life usually seem devoid of pleasure? ☐ Yes ☐ No

Do others view you as eccentric and seclusive? ☐ Yes ☐ No

Do you have a great need for privacy and secrecy? ☐ Yes ☐ No

Do your interests tend toward the abstract, such as science, philosophy and religion? ☐ Yes ☐ No

Do you find it difficult to be warm, tender, and intimate towards others? ☐ Yes ☐ No

Do you have fewer friends than you would like? ☐ Yes ☐ No

Were you considered an introvert as a teenager? ☐ Yes ☐ No

When discouraged, do you often feel apathetic and indifferent? ☐ Yes ☐ No

———————

When confronted with unpredictable disturbances, do you tend to retreat? ☐ Yes ☐ No

Are you often anxious, even when you know you have done your best? ☐ Yes ☐ No

Are you known as a worrier? ☐ Yes ☐ No

Are you often anxious, tense or fearful without knowing why? ☐ Yes ☐ No

Do you have numerous physical complaints which usually do not respond to treatment? ☐ Yes ☐ No

Do you try to help others and then get hurt a lot? ☐ Yes ☐ No

Do you feel that when things go wrong it is usually your fault? ☐ Yes ☐ No

Do you feel guilty when you think others are hurt by your behaviour? ☐ Yes ☐ No

Do you seek intimacy or to be close to others and, yet, shy away from closeness? ☐ Yes ☐ No

Do you frequently feel the need to explain and account for your actions? ☐ Yes ☐ No

Are you more comfortable when you understand "why" things happen? ☐ Yes ☐ No

———————

Do you often lose your temper, and maybe become violent, over seemingly minor things? ☐ Yes ☐ No

Are you an opportunist? ☐ Yes ☐ No

When it comes right down to it, do you think you can beat most people at their own games? ☐ Yes ☐ No

Do you frequently act on impulse and like to take risks? ☐ Yes ☐ No

Do you resist authority figures and enjoy putting them down? ☐ Yes ☐ No

Are you a social non-conformist, a so-called "free soul"? ☐ Yes ☐ No

Do you pride yourself on getting people to do what you want, sometimes without them realizing it? ☐ Yes ☐ No

When you become angry and frustrated, do you tend to do something rather than talk it out? ☐ Yes ☐ No

Do you often do things with little concern about the effects of your behavior? ☐ Yes ☐ No

Do you think that a lot of the feelings that people portray, such as sympathy and compassion, are really kind of silly? ☐ Yes ☐ No

Do others often view your interests and endeavors as unattainable, controversial, or dangerous? ☐ Yes ☐ No

Do you seem to make the same mistake over and over? ☐ Yes ☐ No

Does your family frequently object to the people you go around with? ☐ Yes ☐ No

In general, do people seem not to understand you? ☐ Yes ☐ No

Did you dislike school or consider it a waste of time? ☐ Yes ☐ No

Do you usually tend to gratify your impulses quickly? ☐ Yes ☐ No

Do you often seem to be "in hot water"? ☐ Yes ☐ No

Has your family found more fault with you than you believe you should? ☐ Yes ☐ No

At the same time, we send a small patient information booklet (see Chapter 5) that outlines facts common to all types of cosmetic surgery along with a description of our usual management of rhinoplasty, the risks and usual morbidity involved, and the limitations of the procedure. The booklet and the questionnaire help satisfy the important legal doctrine of informed consent.

Patients are asked to complete the questionnaire at home, preferably with the help of a member of their immediate family or a close friend. This removes at least part of the history-taking process from the office, which some attorneys have claimed is an "emotionally charged atmosphere." It also keeps the collaborating family member or friend informed and, hopefully, secures their approval and cooperation.

Finally, patients are asked to sign and date the form and mail or bring it to the office when they come in for consultation. The legal implications of requiring their signature should be obvious.

The completed form is reviewed with the patient, preferably in the presence of a relative or friend who has accompanied him to the office. Areas in which further investigation seems indicated are probed. Based on the results of the ensuing conversation and physical examination, the patient may be considered (1) an acceptable candidate, (2) a provisionally acceptable candidate depending on the outcome of indicated consultations, or (3) an unacceptable candidate for surgery.

The "Personality Inventory" part of the questionnaire deserves special explanation. Fortunately, most cosmetic surgery patients are not deeply disturbed, nor do they usually present severe reactive problems during the postoperative period. However, experience has shown that some candidates can have notable aberrations that may be easily overlooked by one untrained in detecting cause of psychologic disturbance and in following these leads with care, diligence, and expertise.

The purpose of the inventory, which was developed with the advice of Carl L. Davis, M.D., and Mary R. Wright, Ph.D., is to provide the cosmetic surgeon with a forewarning of the possibility that a substantial psychogenic condition may exist, although such a condition may not be readily apparent. Consultation can then be obtained to probe more deeply into the matter. It is emphasized that this part of the questionnaire is not a diagnostic test and that it does not validate psychopathology. It represents an attempt to "red flag" patterns of psychogenic conditions in patients who are contemplating surgery. It is an impressionistic, not a "scientific" tool.

Basically, three broad areas of psychopathology are dealt with in the inventory: psychoneurotic syndromes, psychosis, and personality disorders. The neurotic patient is recognized by his worry, anxiety, and somatic symptoms; a clue may be gleaned from an unusually large number of affirmative answers the patient has given to questions in the remainder of the questionnaire. The psychotic patient's personality is out of harmony in that his behavior is bizarre, his thoughts are peculiar, and his functioning is deranged. Personality disorders are characterized by behavioral patterns rather than by mental or emotional problems.

Questions in the personality inventory relate to seven types of psychogenic disturbances: depression, hysteria, obsessive-compulsive neurosis, paranoia, and schizoid and psychopathic deviancy. The questions in each section are listed in order of decreasing validity relative to the pattern of the disturbance. The first three or four questions are particularly critical; they are clustered to make the questionnaire easier for the busy surgeon to use and evaluate; affirmative answers to all or most of these are cause for concern, even if all other questions in the section are answered negatively. Of course, the more positive answers one receives, the stronger is the indication for closer observation and for consultation.

5   Preoperative Consultation

It seems to us that the importance of the preoperative management of cosmetic surgery patients has not received the attention it deserves because it is during this period that the seeds of later dissatisfaction are often sown. This is a time when the physician can thoroughly evaluate and educate his patient, establish empathy with him, and institute medicolegal self-protective measures. If done well, both the patient and the physician will come to the operation in the best possible condition and many misunderstandings and untoward incidents can be avoided.

Every surgeon has his own preoperative routine. What we will describe has evolved over a period of time and has served us well.

BEFORE THE FIRST APPOINTMENT

When a patient calls for an appointment, our receptionist determines what type of surgery is sought and three items are mailed to him: a patient education booklet entitled "Cosmetic Surgery" with a covering letter and a Cosmetic Surgery Evaluation Inventory (Fig. 2), which is, as has been previously noted, a self-administered history form.

The letter advises the patient to read the sections of the booklet that pertain to the operation being considered and, then, to complete the history form and return it by mail so that it can be reviewed before the first office visit. Finally, we suggest that they have someone accompany them to the office to buttress the memory of their first consultation because our experience is that persons remember only about one-third of what is told to them preoperatively; later, the friend or relative may help them recall some of the things that they have forgotten.

We have found that the booklet serves several important purposes. It introduces us to patients and establishes the ground rules of the relationship; it helps satisfy their thirst for knowledge while dispelling misconceptions and combatting misinformation; it saves a great deal of our time, yet ensures completeness of disclosure in satisfaction of some of the requirements of the doctrine

of informed consent; it implies thoroughness and serves as a practice-booster in that it is often passed on to others; finally, it reinforces what will be said during the first consultation; it can be reread at any time and can serve as a reference.

In easy-to-understand, nonmedical terms, the booklet discusses the details of the operation, its limitations, the usual morbidity that one can expect, and the risks involved. Also considered are healing dynamics, the maturation of any scars that will ensue, the possibility that the patient might not be satisfied with the results of the operation, and the fact that "touch-up" surgery may be necessary. It stresses that some persons are not good candidates for operation, that the goal of surgery is improvement, not perfection, that no guarantees of results are given or implied, and that one must have acceptable motivations and realistic expectations to be accepted for operation. Finally, the patient is informed of our policy regarding surgical fees and why payment in advance is required. It is stressed that health and hospitalization insurance usually does not cover surgery performed for purely cosmetic reasons and that we will not practice duplicity in an attempt to secure reimbursement for them.

We have already discussed in Chapter 4 why we use a self-administered history questionnaire and what information it provides.

THE FIRST CONSULTATION

Each patient is allotted a 45 minute period on our schedule for the first consultation. When he first checks into the office, a medical record chart is started for him. This is stored in a specially designed manila folder.

Besides containing a section for the usual personal information generally obtained from new patients, our office record form is printed with several diagrams of the head and neck to indicate to the patient where incisions will be placed and, also, to record the locations and configuration of any facial scars or other lesions the patient might have.

On the front cover of the folder is a checklist of the various pre- and postoperative phases of patient management that we deem essential. Its use permits a quick review of whether the different procedures have been carried out without the necessity of hunting through the entire chart for the information.

The new patient is then ushered into a consultation room that, as we have previously mentioned, is comfortable, elegantly furnished, and used only for conferring with preoperative patients. We introduce ourselves in a friendly fashion and exchange a few pleasantries to put the patient at ease before going into the consultation proper.

Young surgeons should appreciate the fact that the patient's first visit is a highly charged emotional affair and often sets the stage for the entire future relationship. The patient is aware of his physical deformity and his subjective distress and, possibly, the social disability it causes him. Furthermore, he has high hopes that surgery will correct this. On the other hand, he is entering an ambience foreign to him, and he often fears that the surgeon may not think his request for change reasonable or possible of fulfillment, that he might be considered vain. There is usually some fear about submitting to surgery and the possibilities of postoperative complications in view of the fact that he is well and free of disease or a life-threatening situation. Then, too, there is concern about the pain, the natural uncertainty about whether or not he will like his new appearance, the attitude of his family and friends to it, and, of course, the cost and affordability of the venture.

On the positive side is the fact that his very presence implies trust in the surgeon's technical competence and professional concern. The physician is established as a powerful therapeutic figure, a dominance that can be retained by proper demeanor, communication, and education.

Next, we review their completed history questionnaire, probe more deeply into areas that their answers indicated potential problems, and conduct a physical examination of the nose externally and internally, if necessary. Then, we take the first of a series of photographs that will become part of the patient's ongoing medical record.

We feel is necessary to digress for a short discussion of office photography. We take all in-office photographs instead of entrusting the task to an office assistant. This ensures less variation in perspective and composition.

The first two photographs, a frontal and lateral view of the patient, is taken with a Polaroid SX-70 camera equipped with a flash bar and a 1.5X telephoto lens to decrease distortion (Fig. 3). The patient is seated in a revolving barstool-type chair set in front of a nonreflecting royal blue background; the chair is centered atop an 8 inch high platform that measures approximately 4 square feet (Fig. 4). We position the patient just as carefully as our medical photographer does; the swivel chair makes it easy to attain and maintain proper positioning.

We find the Polaroid prints useful in a number of ways. They can be used to point out the extent of the deformity; patients are sometimes unaware of this because they seldom have the opportunity of seeing themselves from the side. If they are vague about what they do not like, we simply ask them to point out on the prints what they would like to have corrected. We can show them by means of shading with a black eyebrow pencil what they would like without a nasal hump, with a nose that is shorter or narrower, with a less bulbous tip. The pencil marks can be easily removed so that no permanent record remains. The prints enable us to point out the limitations of

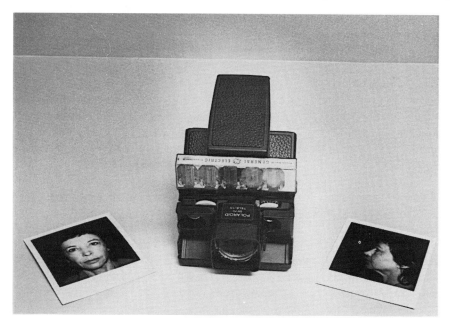

Figure 3. Polaroid SX-70 camera with telephoto lens and the two views of patients taken at their initial visit.

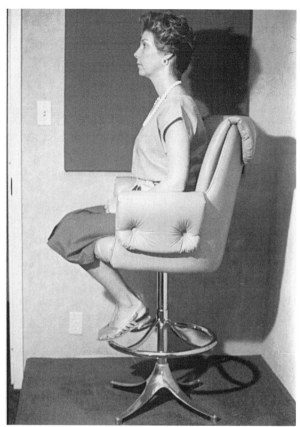

Figure 4.   Rotating stool anchored to elevated dais used when taking office photographs. Background is of non-reflecting royal blue material.

the operation and to demonstrate how foolhardy acceding to some of their requests would be. If a patient becomes "picky" about some aspects of his result during the postoperative period, as some are wont to do, it is very easy to take matching photographs and graphically demonstrate the general improvement that has been achieved.

The Polaroid prints have been helpful in two other ways. By stapling the snapshots inside the front cover of the medical record folder, it becomes easy for us to recall a patient and the extent of his problem if he later telephones to ask questions, no matter how much time has elapsed since his consultation; this is a boon when one has a busy practice and a good memory for faces, but a poor one for names. Finally, when a year has elapsed after the operation, we usually send the referring physician a set of pre- and postoperative views so that he might see the improvement his patient has obtained; they seem to appreciate our thoughtfulness, and the practice has become a good public relations gesture.

At this juncture, we inform the person of any consultations that might be required before we would accept them for operation; these might be with an ophthalmologist, a dermatologist, an internist or cardiologist, a hematologist, a dentist, or a psychiatrist.

We then go into a monologue explaining in a general way the following facts about the procedures they seek: the necessity for obtaining a set of standard medical photographs, where the operation will be performed, procedures at the hospital or the office before the operation, the anesthetic that will be used, the location of the incisions, if any, and the length of time it takes for the scars to mature, the length of time of the operation, the postoperative discomfort and pain, the length of time they will remain in the hospital after the operation, the provision of printed instructions for home care, when they will be expected to return to the office for suture or bandage removal, and, finally, the usual time required for rehabilitation.

Additionally, we advise them not to have the procedure done to please others; not to expect universal recognition of improvement nor approval for what they have done; that the object of every cosmetic operation is improvement, not perfection, and that imperfections might ensue; that they should not expect the surgery to solve any personal problems they might have or change any aspect of their lives or facial features; and that they must have the patience and ego-strength to endure the 1 or 2 weeks of morbidity they can expect.

We discuss the risks they must assume if they wish to undergo surgery. We specifically mention postoperative bleeding and infection, allergy to some medication that will be used, and the possibility of them not being satisfied with the results. We tell them that, in accordance with Louisiana law, we must advise them of serious risks even though they may be scared away from having the operation; then we relate that some of the serious complications known to be associated with any operation, including anesthesia, are death, loss of the function of an organ (and here we mentioned loss of sight, smell, and hearing), paralysis of a member, a stroke, and disfiguring scars. To soften the blow somewhat, we tell them that the chance of these disasters occurring are small, but add that they do exist.

We have available several books containing pre- and postoperative photographs of patients who have had the various operations, but we use them selectively. Some unsophisticated patients ask to see what can be accomplished; others want to be convinced that the resultant scars will usually be almost imperceptible and easily covered by makeup. We also use them to point out imperfections that may be present after the operation, the necessity for using implants in some cases, and the relationship of the reconstructed nose to other facial features.

We are well aware of the arguments against

using photographs of other patients for demonstration, particularly those relating to implied warranty and invasion of privacy. So, we always preface the use of a picture book with statements to the effect that it is not a catalog from which a nose can be chosen, nor will their result be the same as those pictured. We stress that they are being shown the pictures simply to demonstrate some facts about the operation, that no warranty is being given or implied. Likewise, we would not use the picture of any patient without their written permission, for this would indeed constitute invasion of privacy. Incidentally, we also sometimes use photographs of patients to demonstrate the extent of the morbidity that occasionally follows some operations.

Each practitioner has to decide for himself whether or not to use pre- and postoperative photographs for patient education purposes. We concede that their use is debatable but feel that they can be of inestimable value if used judiciously; for example, we would infinitely prefer to have a candidate for operation forego the procedure because of revulsion caused by a photograph than to have him later accuse us of not informing him of exactly what he was getting into. It should be emphasized that these books of photographs are not scattered through the office to try to impress patients or to "sell" operations; we use them for patient education purposes only.

Following this, we inquire if the patient has any additional questions. Usually, our exposé has been so thorough that they have little further to ask other than the cost of their operation. We provide them with this information, along with an estimate of hospital charges, on a form that provides a resumé of the consultation in the event that they forget some of the details.

At the end of the consultation, if the patient wants to pursue the matter of having surgery, we order any indicated consultations, advise them to see our medical photographer if there are no contraindications to the operation uncovered by the consultants, and schedule a second consultation with them at a later date. On the other hand, the patient may wish to give the matter further consideration or seek a second opinion; incidentally, we view the first visit as being exploratory on the patient's part and never pressure him to "sign up." In either case, they are invited to telephone us if they have any further questions.

THE SECOND CONSULTATION

The second consultation is scheduled after the patient's photographs have been received from the medical photographer; usually, there is a week's interval between the two consultations. This gives the patient time to formulate further questions to allay his concerns and gives us time to study the case at further length and plan its execution.

When the patient arrives for the consultation, the photographic prints are displayed for inspection, and he is given some time alone to examine them in the privacy of the consultation room. After a reasonable period, we join him to discuss the deformities the photographs reveal and describe the goals of the proposed correction. We speak in terms of what we will try to accomplish and point out the inherent limitations of the operation. We encourage further questions and attempt to answer them satisfactorily.

Having done all we possibly could do from the standpoint of patient education, we now ask for a commitment. If the patient decides to go ahead with the operation, we help him select a suitable date and, then, complete a number of additional preparatory steps.

First, we take a set of 35 mm Kodachrome transparencies in the standard position; these become part of the medical record and are kept in plastic sheets in the patient's medical record folder. We use Kodachrome 64 film and a single lens reflex 35 mm Nikon camera with a pentaprism viewfinder and a 105 mm micro lens (Fig. 5); this permits an ideal camera-to-subject distance of about 4 feet and allows adequate depth of focus. An electronic flash attached to the camera provides adequate light to compensate for a rather small lens opening.

Several test rolls of film should be exposed by using various f-stops to establish the optimum exposure; once established, these settings should always be used for the sake of uniformity. Frontal and lateral views of the entire head are taken with the horizontal format of the film held in a vertical position; the horizontal format of the film is used for the basal view.

The center of the camera viewfinder should be level with the Frankfort horizontal line; the barrel of the lens should be perpendicular to the frontal or sagittal planes of the head, depending on the views being taken; and the film should parallel the same planes.

When a frontal view is taken, the camera-to-subject distance should be adjusted until the head almost fills the viewfinder (125 cm, or 52 inches, with our lens) and is centered so that equal amounts of each ear show on each side to avoid rotation, and the forehead hairline and mandible are equidistant from the top and bottom edges, respectively.

In lateral views, the ear should be included and the eyelashes and eyebrows should be aligned so that those away from the camera cannot be seen;

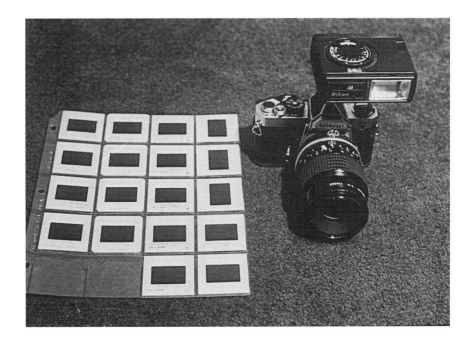

Figure 5. Nikon camera with a 105 mm microlens used to take Kodachrome transparencies before and after the operation. Slides are stored in the patient's chart in plastic sheets.

neither should the half of the philtrum nearest the background be visible.

The camera-to-subject distance for our basal view is 52 cm. The eyes should be centered and the nasal tip should be superimposed over the nasal dorsum when the basal view is taken.

After the Kodachrome transparancies have been taken, we complete our standard consent form (Fig. 1) in a manner appropriate for the patient and sign it. Next, we ask the patient to read it in the presence of our scheduling assistant and offer to answer any questions inspired by the completed form. We do not personally read the form to them, as is sometimes recommended, because they have been exposed to its contents at least three times: when they read the Cosmetic Surgery booklet before the first consultation, during our first consultation, and while completing their history questionnaire. If there are no further questions after reading the form, the patient is required to sign it, and his signature is witnessed by an assistant. Incidentally, our signed consent forms are not kept in the medical record folder. Since we had one mysteriouly disappear from the folder of a patient who later filed suit, we store them separately.

The consent form having been signed, the scheduling assistant then provides the patient with several items:

1. Instructions to be followed before hospital admission. These are time savers and serve to eliminate much confusion and many telephone calls.

2. A confirmation of surgical arrangements form to be read and signed. Essentially, these forms indicate where the surgery will be performed, what time the patient should report, that we will request the accommodations they desire, although we cannot guarantee their availability, what the surgical fee will be, when the payment is due, and, finally, the fact that the surgical fee does not cover the hospital charge.

3. A pamphlet containing postoperative instructions. Again, this has proved to be a time saver and ensures that the patient receives all the instructions needed; it helps those assisting in his postoperative care at home.

4. Four prescriptions, two to be used before the operation and the remainder afterward. We prescribe citrobioflavinoids and anti-inflammatory enzymes before surgery; our clinical impression is that they help to decrease operative bleeding and postoperative edema. A few sedatives and mild analgesics are prescribed for use during the early postoperative period.

Finally, before the patient leaves the office, he is advised to telephone us if he wishes further information and to inform us immediately if he develops any type of infection in the immediate preoperative period.

6 Planning Rhinoplasty

Rhinoplastic surgeons undertake one of the most demanding operations in plastic surgery on the most visible part of the body. The nose that a surgeon creates will be on permanent public display for the remainder of the patient's life. This is an awesome responsibility with far-reaching implications, ranging from the patient's satisfaction to public judgment of the surgeon's skill. It follows then that each operation should be planned in advance if one wants to achieve the highest general average of good results.

Successful planning presupposes a knowledge of what are considered ideal nasal and facial proportions. This can be learned from the artist. With such a background, the surgeon can determine what the ideal nose for his patient would be and set the goal for the operation. Good photographs become an indispensable part of the planning process.

FACIAL PROPORTIONS

Francis Bacon said, "There is no excellent beauty which hath not some strangeness of proportion." This was established long ago by the ancient Egyptians, who were the first to use arithmetic in art. They found that their structures, sculpture, and painting were more interesting and pleasing if construction was based on carefully worked out geometry and proportions; as a result, the so-called golden proportion became the basis of their concept of beauty. It is that division of a line in which the smaller part is the same proportion to the greater part as the greater part is to the whole.

Eudoxus, the Greek mathematician, worked out the mathematics of the golden proportion and found that it could be expressed as a formula that has since been widely used in architecture and in art. Pythagoras, the Greek geometer, discovered that this formula could also be the basis for the proportions of the human figure. He showed that the human body is built with each part in definite proportions to all other parts.

Leonardo da Vinci, like Pythagoras, made a close study of the human figure and also demonstrated how all of its different parts were related in the golden proportion. He taught that the face should be divided into three equal horizontal spaces, the upper third consisting of the forehead, the middle third occupied by the nose, and the lower third extending from the nasolabial angle to the chin. He also showed how these areas were further subdivided into spaces that are occupied by other features (the eyes, the upper lips, the ears) in such a way that there is a high degree of proportional regularity.

PHOTOGRAPHIC ANALYSIS

Visual inspection gives only a general idea of the nasal deformity, so facial analysis is best accomplished, in our opinion, by studying a set of preoperative photographs taken in a standardized manner. Early in our career we used wax casts and dental stone, but making them is time-consuming and expensive, and they offer little or no advantage over a good set of photographs.

A suitable set of photographs for rhinoplasty consists of a frontal view, two lateral views, and one view of the base of the nose (Fig. 6). Many surgeons use an additional lateral view taken with the patient smiling. The frontal and profile views should be one-half life size, and the basal view life size. Contact prints measuring 5 by 7 inches are preferable. Posing, composition, lighting, and printing should always conform to rigid standards; faults detract from reliability for analysis and diagnosis.

We use the services of a medical photographer who understands our needs as far as uniformity and standardization are concerned. He uses a view camera having a 105 mm lens and provides two sets of glossy black and white prints that we use to plan the operation and in the operating room, and for publication illustrations.

The main landmark used for photographing a patient before rhinoplasty is the Frankfort horizontal line; it connects the upper rim of the external auditory canal to the lower rim of the bony orbit. This line should be absolutely horizontal in both frontal and lateral views.

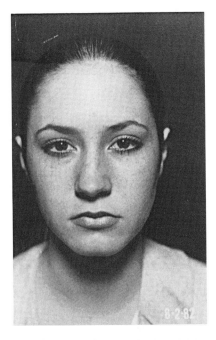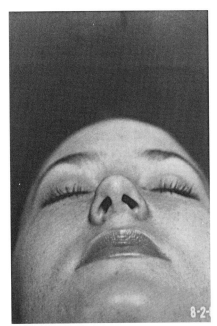

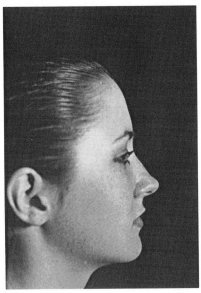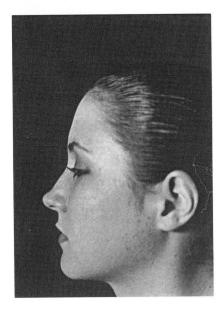

Figure 6. Standard set of rhinoplasty photographs.

The midline of the face is determined by constructing a line that connects the center of the forehead at the hairline, the nasion, a point at the root of the nasal spine (the subnasale), and the anterior point of the mental symphysis (the gnathion). This line should be perpendicular to the floor and to the Frankfort horizontal line (Fig. 7).

Several guides are helpful in determining the "trueness" of the views. In a true lateral pose, for example, no portion of the eyebrow nearest the background should be seen; likewise, only one of the ridges of the philtrum should be visible. Very little of the forehead should be seen in the basal view lest there be a foreshortening of the columella.

Rarely are the two halves of a face symmetrical. This is well-recognized by actors and actresses; some actually refuse to be photographed from certain angles lest their "bad side" be seen. Neither is it uncommon to find one eyebrow or eye higher than the other, nor one cheek and jawbone more prominent than the other. The lips are frequently slanted. Even the Cupid's bow of the upper lip may be off to one side, so it cannot be depended on to determine the midline of the face.

Asymmetries should be pointed out to the patient before the operation for several reasons. First, an adequately straightened nose sometimes appears somewhat deviated because of the patient's underlying facial imbalance. Also, patients complain about one side of the operated nose

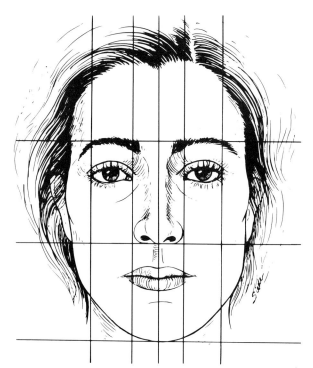

Figure 7. The midline of the face, a line connecting the center of the forehead at the hairline, the nasion, and the subnasale perpendicular to the Frankfort horizontal line. The face is divided into equal vertical components based on the intercanthal distances.

looking better than the other when such is not the case; it may be due to the contour and structure of that side of the face. Finally, some patients erroneously ascribe changes in the remainder of the face to the effects of rhinoplasty, for example, a straightened nose may cause one-half of the face to appear fuller.

AESTHETIC NORMS

When studying the patient's nose and face before the operation and planning the changes he would like to make, the surgeon should keep in mind certain relationships to determine whether the nose being considered harmonizes with the remainder of the face and head.

Assuming that the patient has been posed correctly, a beginner can conveniently plot facial measurements by placing a print of a standard frontal view face forward on the glass surface of a lighted x-ray view box, a window pane, or some other strong light source and drawing horizontal and vertical lines on the back surface of the print to divide the face into its various components.

The width of each eye is the primary measurement used in dividing the face into its vertical components (Fig. 7). If vertical lines are drawn parallel to the midline at each medial and lateral

canthus and also at points one eye's width lateral to the outer canthi, the face should be divided into five equal parts. The horizontal proportions of the face are established by drawing lines perpendicular to the midline at four points: the trichion, the nasion, the subnasale, and the gnathion. This should provide three equal horizontal segments.

The ala nasi should be of the same width as the middle vertical space. The nasal dorsum should be one-half as wide, and the width of the lobule should occupy two-thirds of the space. The midline of the nose should correspond to the midline of the face; otherwise, the two sides will be asymmetrical.

The nose should extend the entire length of the middle horizontal division of the face. Ideally, no more than one-third of the vertical height of the nostrils should be visible when the nose is viewed from the front. Frontal views establish the symmetry of the two sides, as well as the length and width, of the face.

The lateral views should be used to study the length and contour of the nasal dorsum and its projection from the face, the amount of lobular projection, the status of the nasolabial and nasofrontal angles, the type of forehead, chin, and mid-third of the face that the patient has, the general direction of the lateral crura and long axes of the nostrils, the contour and inclination of the columella and its relationship to the alar margins, and, finally, the comparative heights of the columella and upper lip. Incidentally, it will be found that in lateral views, the base of the ear falls almost on the same line as the base of the nose.

If one constructs a vertical line connecting the most prominent point of the forehead with the most prominent portion of the chin, it should pass near a point midway between the alar-facial and nasolabial angles and close to the vermilion border of the lower lip. The point of the chin should be near or should touch that line; the nasofrontal angle should lie on or just below the line; finally, the line is used to plot the angle at which the nose projects from the face (Fig. 8). An angle somewhere between 30° and 38° is generally considered pleasing, depending on the projection of the remaining elements of the profile.

To determine columella inclination, a vertical line that is perpendicular to the Frankfort horizontal line and passes through the alar-facial angle is constructed. Another line is then drawn through the long axes of the nostrils, and the angle formed by the transecting lines is measured (Fig. 9). A nasolabial angle of 90° to 105° in women, depending on their height and chin projection, is normal. Incidentally, the nasolabial angle should

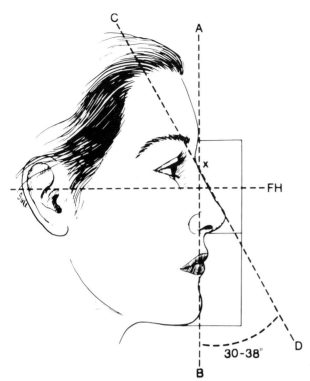

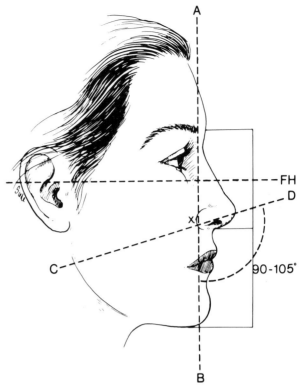

Figure 8. Determining nasal projection. AB, a line connecting the most prominent parts of the forehead and chin; it should pass midway between the alar-facial and nasolabial angles and close to the vermilion border of the lower lip, and also be perpendicular to the Frankfort horizontal (FH) line. CD, a line along the nasal dorsum should describe an angle of 30°–38° with line AB.

Figure 9. A method of determining columellar inclination. FH, a line passing through the alar-facial angle and perpendicular to the Frankfort horizontal line. CD, a line passing through the long axis of the nostrils. The angle should be from 90° to 95° in men and from 95° to 105° in women, depending on other profile characteristics.

lie 2 to 3 mm below the alar-facial angle; if less, it is considered retracted; if more, "webbing" is said to exist.

As previously mentioned, many surgeons require a profile view taken when the patient is smiling because certain deformities become obvious or exaggerated only during smiling. For example, a nose whose dorsum is straight during repose may present a convexity during smiling, or the converse may be true. Webbing of the nasolabial angle or "crowding" of the upper lip may appear. The alae may flare excessively or their bases may move so high that too much of the columella, or even the nasal septum, becomes visible.

The basal view demonstrates the size, shape, and symmetry of the nostrils, the width, length, and possible deviations of the columella, the ratio between columellar length and height of the lobule, and the thickness and contour of the alae. Information is also provided about the length of the medial crura and the possibility of a deflection of the caudal end of the septum. Ideally, the base of the nose should resemble an equilateral triangle, the length of the columella being twice the height of the lobule and equal to the length of the upper

lip; the nostrils should be pear-shaped and about the same width as the columella (Fig. 10).

PLANNING THE CORRECTION

After the deformity has been analyzed on the photographs and its relationship to the other facial components considered, the goal of the operation can be established. Obviously, the aim should be to bring the abnormality within the range of the norm for the particular individual.

This approach provides surgical direction with a rational basis. The practice of undertaking an operation with only a preliminary visual examination is, in our opinion, to be unequivocally condemned; the patient deserves better.

Help in establishing the goal of surgery can be obtained by pencil shading the parts of the nose to be altered on the reverse side of the black and white 5 by 7 inch preoperative photographs that have been placed face forward on a lighted view box (Fig. 11).

Our first step is to try to determine what the ideal length of the nasal dorsum would be for the face of the patient in question; this is the distance

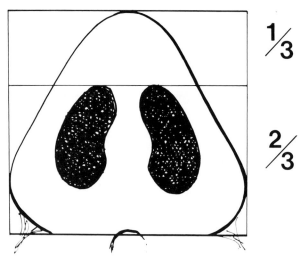

Figure 10. Basal view aesthetics. The base of the nose should resemble an equilateral triangle. The length of the columella should be twice the height of the lobule and equal to the length of the upper lip. The nostrils should be pear-shaped, and each nostril should be approximately the width of the columella.

from the nasofrontal angle to the tip of the lobule. Because a reciprocal relationship exists between the length of the dorsum and the nasolabial angle, this parameter is simultaneously established when the new dorsal length is planned.

Because our goal is to recontour the nasal pyramid so that it makes an angle of approximately 35° to 38° with the facial plane, the next step is to establish where the tip of the lobule should be, in view of the newly established dorsal length. The depth of the nasofrontal angle must also be considered; it should be located about 15 mm above the level of the medial canthi.

When these two important points, the desired projection of the tip of the nose and the depth of the nasofrontal angle, have been established, one need only plot a line between them to determine how much the hump must be leveled or how much the dorsum has to be augmented.

Finally, from a study of the frontal and basal views, one can decide how much the bony pyramid, the lobule, and the alae must be modified.

The photographs are always taken to the operating room, where they are placed in a special holder so that they can be referred to from time to time during the procedure.

ADDITIONAL CONSIDERATIONS IN THE PLANNING PROCEDURE

There are a number of additional facts of importance that should be kept in mind when planning a rhinoplasty:

1. A disproportion of one feature is generally not as bad as of two features, for example, a hump nose in conjunction with underdevelopment of the chin. Both deformities should be corrected for an optimal result. We feel strongly that a surgeon is justified in refusing to operate on a person who refuse simultaneous chin augmentation.

2. Although most people seeking rhinoplasty want a change in the size or contour of the entire nose, some seek to change only one area, for example, a bulbous tip. Partial rhinoplasty is rarely wise, and the results will prove, as a rule, aesthetically disappointing.

3. Small changes are more difficult to make and require more precision than large ones because the margin for error is smaller. The visible improvement obtained will also be smaller.

4. Gross reductions should be approached carefully, since there is a definite limit to how much a nose can be reduced in size; in addition, such patients may have difficulty adjusting to markedly smaller noses.

5. The factors that limit surgical execution and therefore achievement of the surgical goal should be kept in mind. These include excessive thickness and oiliness of the skin, which may limit contractility, an increase in the amount of subcutaneous tissue that has the same effect, the amount of previous trauma sustained by the nose, and the need for considerable simultaneous septal work.

6. Patients with wide faces should have well-defined nasal bridges and noses that are not too small; likewise, one should be careful not to make the nose too short for patients who have long faces.

7. Tall individuals should not have too much columellar tilt because too much of the nostrils will show and the alae may look too wide. On the other hand, women can tolerate more columellar tilt than men.

8. A prominent chin calls for a straight dorsum and a nasolabial angle of no more than 95°, whereas a "soft" chin will permit more columellar inclination and more of a *retroussé* effect; however, in general, if the chin is "soft", and the nose is already short, a straight dorsum is generally more pleasing.

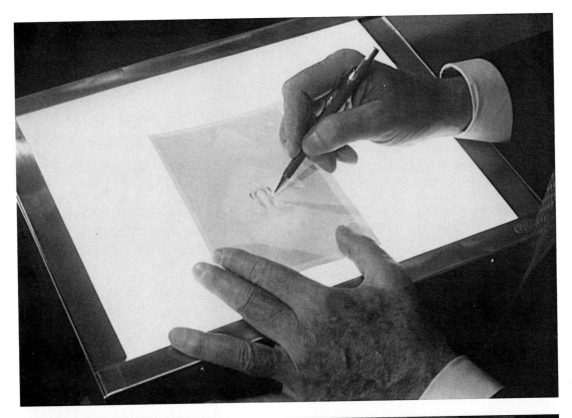

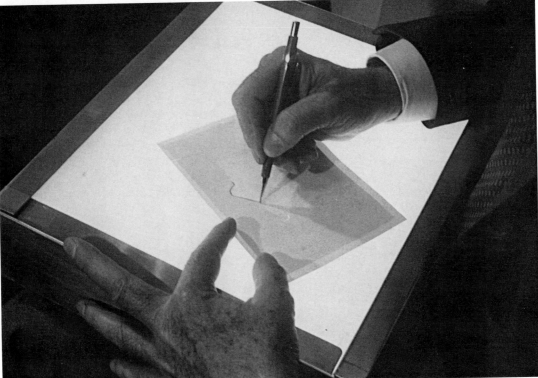

Figure 11.   Top: Indicating proposed changes in frontal view on the back of preoperative photograph. Bottom: Planning changes in dorsal contour and length on back of profile view.

9. One should be careful when removing a hump and shortening the nose of a patient whose forehead slants; such persons must have adequate chin projection, a well-defined nasofrontal angle, and a straight, rather than concave, dorsum.

10. The dorsum should also be straight if there is an increased forward tilt of the upper lip due to excessive projection of the teeth.

11. The tip of the nose should show three planes when viewed in profile: dorsal, columellar, and a slanting plan connecting the two. Furthermore, the aesthetic effect seems more pleasing when the high point of the tip projects 1 or 2 mm above the level of the cartilagenous dorsum.

12. Tip recession often causes increased convexity of the alae, particularly of their bases; correction of this condition may have to be included in the operation.

13. The corrected nose must look good from the frontal view; after all, this is the view from which most noses are seen by others. Unfortunately, many who have had rhinoplasties have wider noses after the operation than before; this is painfully apparent in too many articles in the medical literature.

14. When medical photographs are taken, it is important that a patient's hairstyle not interfere with the exposure of various divisions of the face; use of a head band similar to those commonly used by tennis players will obviate this.

7   Topographic and Surgical Anatomy

TOPOGRAPHY

Although it is necessary to establish terms of reference at the start of any discussion, it is particularly important with respect to the nose. No other area of the body is subjected to so much conflicting and confusing terminology as far as position and direction are concerned. This is largely due to the tendency of some surgeons to switch designations when the patient changes from an erect to a supine position.

In anatomic discussions, the body is always assumed to be in the erect position and face forward, and the terms of relationships are used strictly with reference to this position. These terms should not be changed when the position of the body is changed. Thus, the terms "cephalic" and "caudal" correspond to superior and inferior, respectively, and "ventral" and "dorsal" to anterior and posterior (Fig. 12).

The line at which a vertical or sagittal plane meets the surface of the nose to divide it into similar and nearly equal halves will be called the "midline." The words "medial" and "lateral" will denote nearer or farther from the midline, respectively. "Internal" will refer to surfaces within the nasal cavity, whereas "external" will indicate the outer surface of the nasal structure. "Superficial" and "deep" refer to depth from the surface. Each nasal cavity will be spoken of as having a "roof," a "floor," and "septal" and "lateral" walls.

Sometimes, popular usage will cause a descriptive term to become so deeply ingrained that it must be accepted even though it might prove confusing and offensive to purists. Such a term is "nasal dorsum," which is commonly accepted to mean the rounded median ridge of the external nose (Fig. 13). It has become a fact of life that must be accepted, so much so that the use of the term "nasal ventrum" would seem awkward.

The external nose resembles a pyramid, apex upward, one of whose surfaces is attached to the face; the other two meet to form the aforementioned nasal dorsum, or "bridge," of the nose whose caudal limit is the "nasal tip."

The area of the forehead located between the eyebrows is known as the "glabella." The "nasofrontal angle" is the angle formed between the external nose and the forehead; it may vary from shallow, as in certain works of Greek sculpture, such as the Venus de Milo, to deep, as in saddle nose deformities and in many Asians. The "nasion" is a point in the nasofrontal angle that corresponds to the midpoint of the nasofrontal suture line. The cephalic portion of the nose, where the pyramid emerges from the forehead, is called the "radix nasi" or "root" of the nose; it is also sometimes referred to as the "subglabellar segment."

One-third to one-half of the nasal dorsum is called the "bony dorsum" because it is formed by the confluence of the two nasal bones; the remainder is called the "cartilagenous dorsum" or "septal dorsum," since it is composed of septal cartilage. The "rhinion" is the name given to the junction of the bony and cartilagenous parts of the nasal bridge, and the region just cephalic to the nasal tip is termed the "supratip area."

Strictly speaking, the area of the nasal pyramid formed by the conjoined lower lateral cartilages is the "base of the nose," not the "tip." The "tip" is the free angle formed by the rounding of the medial and lateral crura (Fig. 14).

The base of the nose is triangular in outline when viewed from below. That part above the level of the nostrils is the "lobule." The lobule, like the entire base of which it is a part, is supposed to be triangular in outline, its apex being the tip of the nose. The portion of the lobule located between the tip and the upper border of the nostrils is known as the "infratip lobule." The remaining two-thirds of the base contains two pear-shaped openings, or nostrils, that are separated by a bridge of tissue, the "columella." The lateral walls of the nostrils are the "alae." They usually curve medially toward the base of the columella to form rolls of tissue called the "sills" of the nostrils.

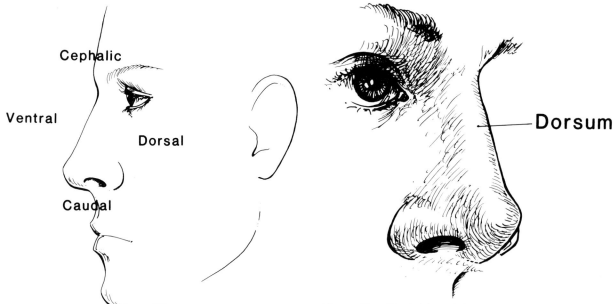

Figure 12. Terms used to describe nasal relationships.

Figure 13. The bridge of the nose is commonly referred to as the nasal dorsum instead of nasal ventrum.

The area above the incisor teeth and below the nostrils is referred to as the "premaxillary area," and the angle between the columella and the upper lip is known as the "nasolabial angle" or "subnasale."

Two important features of the nasal base are the "external soft tissue triangles," sometimes loosely referred to as "facets" because, in some cases, they may give the area a sculptured appearance. Located just above the apices of the nostrils, they are composed of webs of soft tissue that bridge the gap between the caudal margins of the medial and lateral crural cartilages within

the lobule. A similar arrangement exists at the lobular end of the membranous septum but is, of course, not visible unless the nostril margins are retracted; these are the "internal soft tissue triangles." Their importance lies in the fact that an imaginary line drawn between the apices of the internal and external soft triangles will mark the junction of the medial and lateral crura of each alar cartilage; this is called the "angle of the lower lateral cartilage" and should not be confused with the "dome of the vestibule." The latter is the highest part of the vestibule and is formed mainly by the undersurface of the medial ends of the

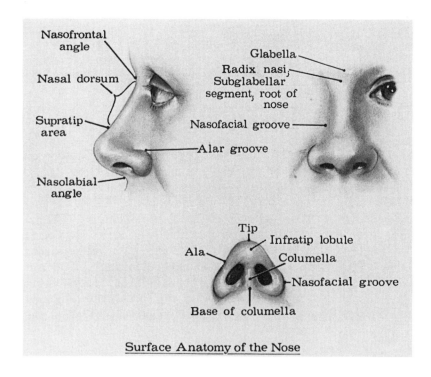

Surface Anatomy of the Nose

Figure 14. Surface landmarks of the nose.

lateral crura. The grooves that mark the attachment of the lateral walls of the nose to the face are known as the "nasofacial grooves," and where the alae meet the face, they become the "alar-facial grooves." Superiorly, the nasofacial grooves become the "jugonasal grooves." Finally, the two furrows that begin at the alar-facial grooves and continue downward laterally to the corners of the mouth are called the "melolabial grooves." The furrows that divide the alae from the remainder of the lateral nasal walls are known as the "alar-nasal grooves."

SURGICAL ANATOMY

Soft Tissue Covering

The scanty attention given the soft tissue covering of the nose belies its importance in aesthetic rhinoplasty. Its thickness varies; normally, it is thickest overlying the radix and in the supratip area, and thinnest at the rhinion (Fig. 15). This arrangement serves to smooth out the depressions and prominences of the nasal skeleton. Thus, the soft tissues can produce part of the primary deformity, and one must compensate for soft tissue thickness when modifying the nose.

Shallowness of the nasofrontal angle can be caused by part of the procerus muscle that spans the area. Wideness of the same muscle or the corrugators can produce a broadness of the same area.

The relative denseness of the supratip soft tissue is due mainly to thick epithelium that contains more than the usual amount of oil glands and an increased amount of subcutaneous tissue; fibers of the compressor naris muscle are encountered lateral to the midline. When too thick, these tissues become inelastic and will not conform to the remodeled framework unless special measures are taken.

The thinness of the tissues at the rhinion indicates that it is the highest point of the skeletal profile in a good-looking nose; from that point, the skeletal profile slants in both directions. This condition must be recreated at the end of the operation.

Skeleton of the External Nose

As previously mentioned, the external nose resembles a pyramid. Approximately the upper half is composed of bone. The lower half consists of cartilage, but the proportions may vary.

Descending from the forehead, the bony skeleton consists of the nasal part of the frontal bone, the medially paired nasal bones, and the two frontal processes of the maxillary bones posterolateral to them. These bones constitute the bony vault of the nose (Fig. 16).

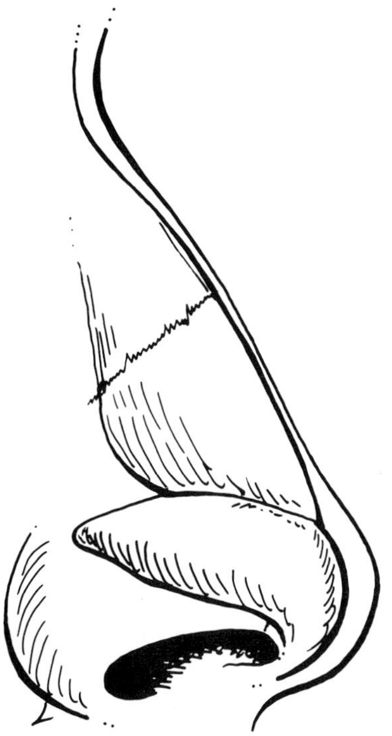

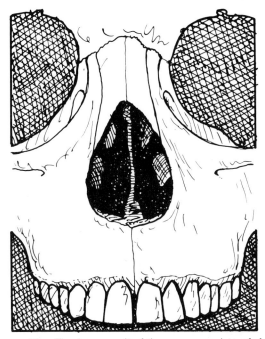

Figure 15.   Relative thickness of the soft tissues covering the skeleton along the dorsum of the nose; they are thinnest at the rhinion.

Figure 16.   The bony vault of the nose consists of, from above downward, the nasal process of the frontal bone, the paired nasal bones centrally and the two frontal processes of the maxillary bones posterolateral to the nasal bones.

On the anterior aspect of the dried skull, the free margins of the frontal processes outline a pear-shaped opening, the piriform aperture; through it, one can see the two cavities of the internal nose and their intervening septum. During life, the cartilagenous elements of the external nasal skeleton almost fill the piriform opening. These consist of the ventral margin of the septal cartilage in the midline, the paired upper lateral cartilages attached to it, and the lower lateral or alar cartilages. The cephalic margins of the upper laterals extend a few millimeters under the nasal bones and adjacent parts of the frontal processes; their lateral ends do not reach the piriform margins but are attached to them by thick fibrous tissue; their caudal ends always terminate 4 to 6 mm proximal to the superior septal angle and are overlapped by the cephalic margins of the alar cartilages.

Sometimes, the cartilagenous portion of the nasal skeleton is said to be composed of upper and lower cartilagenous vaults. The upper vault consists of the two upper lateral cartilages. The lower vault is composed of the two lower lateral cartilages that give form to the base of the nose.

Nasal Bones

The paired nasal bones articulate with each other to form the bridge of the nose and are attached to the frontal bone above. The unit they form is narrow and strong at the root of the nose,

or radix nasi; in fact, this is the strongest part of the nasal skeleton, and it takes great force to fracture the area. The strength stems from the fact that the upper ends of the bones are solid in cross-section (Fig. 17) and form a mortise joint by surrounding the frontal spine; in addition, they derive support from the underlying bony septum, but this is not critical in maintaining their projection.

The dense upper portions of the conjoint bones taper as they proceed caudally; the tentlike structure they describe becomes wider, and its walls become thinner. This accounts for the frequency of fractures in these relatively weak areas.

An interesting point is that the thick tapered core of the combined bones acts as a fulcrum and determines the site and direction of fracture when lateral force is applied to narrow the nose during rhinoplasty. This can be readily and invariably demonstrated in cadaveric specimens and refutes the depiction of the location and direction of superior osteotomy in so many texts and articles on rhinoplasty.

The narrowness and density of the bones in the radix nasi contradicts another long-standing teaching and practice concept, namely, that medial osteotomies must be carried up to the frontal bone if one desires to narrow the nasal pyramid. In the first place, the radix area rarely needs narrowing, so it need not be invaded as a rule. Secondly, the kerf created in the dense bone by the osteotome will hardly permit narrowing; it would be necessary to remove intervening bone or shave the outer surfaces to do that.

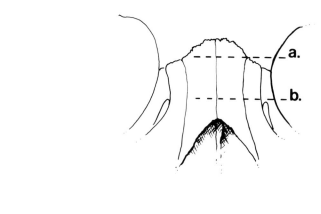

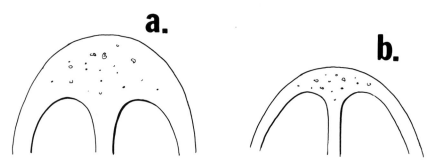

Figure 17. Relative thickness of the nasal bones at two levels. They are thick above (a), where they form part of the radix, and thin below (b).

It is important to remember that the caudal ends of the nasal bones overlap the cephalic borders of the upper cartilagenous vault for a short distance, so the upper laterals should be cut from the septum in this area when narrowing the nose.

The structure of the undersurface of the bones is of interest. It presents a crest formed by the inner extension of each medial border that articulates with the underlying septum. The crest resembles the prow of a ship in that it narrows as it proceeds caudally. This means that the roof of the nasal cavity veers slightly lateralward in this area, a fact of importance when medial osteotomies are performed.

Frontal Processes of the Maxillae

These structures form the remainder of each side wall of the nose and determine the width of the piriform opening and the form and dimensions of the nose. They abut the nasal and frontal bones and are relatively thick where they meet the remainder of the maxillae at the nasofacial groove but become thinner and narrower in their upper reaches.

Lateral osteotomies begin in the grooves at the level of the anterior ends of the inferior turbinates and extend upward as far as the nasal process of the frontal bone.

Upper Lateral Cartilages

These two flat triangular plates occupy the middle third of the nose and form the upper cartilagenous vault. Medially, they and their covering mucoperichondrium are continuous with the septum. Superiorly, they are overlapped by the caudal borders of the nasal bones, and their inferior ends are overlapped by the lateral crura (Fig. 18). Laterally, they do not extend to the piriform margins, the hiatus being filled with strong fibrous tissue.

The angle they make with the septal cartilage is most acute, on the order of 10°, at their inferior ends; this is called the valve area. The angle enlarges above because the septal dorsum widens. Scar tissue or cartilagenous deformities in this area may hinder breathing.

The caudal ends of the upper laterals end 4 to 6 mm cephalic to the superior septal angle. If septal length is shortened, the caudal ends must also be shortened. Otherwise, they will protrude into the vestibule. Sometimes they curve outward and contribute to the wideness of the nasal dorsum and lateral walls in the area.

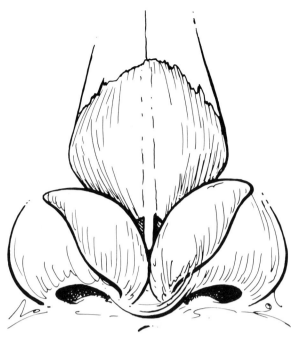

Figure 18.   The upper lateral cartilages. Their cephalic ends extend beneath the nasal bones for a distance of a few millimeters; their caudal ends are overlapped by the scrolls of the lateral crura.

Lower Lateral Cartilages

Each alar cartilage surrounds the upper part of the nostril and consists of a medial and lateral crus that is continuous at a point called the angle. The lateral crus complex (crus plus attached sesamoid or accessory cartilages) is always longer than the medial crus and extends to the piriform aperature; since it is located at a level higher than the medial crus, each alar cartilage resembles a slightly sprung horseshoe. The medial crura extend for varying distances into the columella, and their free ends usually overlap a portion of the caudal end of the septal cartilage.

The alar cartilages have important soft tissue connections with the septal cartilage, the upper lateral cartilages, and each other; along with the flexibility of the septal cartilage, this arrangement permits considerable movement of the nasal base. It should be noted that the lower margins of these cartilages do not extend to the free edges of the nostrils except in part of the columella. The detailed surgical anatomy of these cartilages will be considered in Chapter 11 when nasal base surgery is discussed.

Nasal Septum

The surgical anatomy of the nasal septum will be considered in detail in Chapter 12 when correction of that structure is considered.

8 Premedication and Anesthesia

We use local anesthesia almost exclusively. If there are no medical contraindications, we feel a properly used local anesthetic offers several distinct advantages to the rhinoplastic surgeon: it is safer, it reduces operative bleeding, it does not render the patient unconscious so that he can cooperate if necessary, and, finally, it is cheaper, not a small consideration in this era of ever-rising medical costs.

A prerequisite for local anesthesia is adequate premedication. This can be achieved with a combination of drugs, each of which plays a specific role in allaying the patient's apprehension, elevating the pain threshold, reducing reflex irritability, producing amnesia, and counteracting possible undesirable effects of the anesthetic agent. Our aim is to have hospitalized patients arrive in the operating room in a somnolent but arousable and cooperative state. Less preanesthetic medication is used when office surgery is to be done.

PREANESTHETIC MEDICATION ROUTINE

Our premedication routine is as follows:

Three hours before surgery:

Adults are given 200 mg of pentobarbital (Nembutal) orally; teenagers are given 100 mg.

Two hours before surgery:

Both adults and teenagers are given an additional 100 mg of pentobarbital orally plus 100 mg of dimenhydrinate (Dramamine).

One hour before surgery:

Patients weighing more than 125 lb are given 2 mg of hydromorphone hydrochloride (Dilaudid) intramuscularly; those weighing less than 125 lb receive 1 mg; in addition, all patients receive 0.16 mg of scopolamine intramuscularly.

The pentobarbital component of the regimen is designed to allay anxiety, to depress the central nervous system, and to antagonize the possible toxic effects of the local anesthetic agent.

Dimenhydrinate is a safe drug with few contraindications. It causes mild drowsiness, dries secretions, and is effective in the prevention of nausea and vomiting caused by the subsequent use of opiates.

Hydromorphone hydrochloride is a potent analgesic, eight times more potent on a milligram basis than morphine, which in turn is eight times more potent and causes less respiratory depression than meperidine (Demerol).

The small dose of scopolamine (0.16 mg) dries secretions, depresses vagal nerve reflexes, produces amnesia, and provides greater neutralization of respiratory depression than atropine. Scopolamine has a bad reputation because it causes excitement, restlessness, hallucinations, or delirium, although rarely. We have experienced few such reactions over the past 30 years from the small dosage we use; these were easily reversible with physostigmine (Antilirium).

Most of our patients arrive at the operating room in the desired condition, that is, somnolent but arousable; this permits us to proceed with injection of the local anesthetic without further delay. If they are still "awake" or exhibit anxiety about the imminent local anesthetic injection, we usually find that the intravenous administration of 1 or 2 mg of diazepam (Valium) or droperidol (Inapsine) will provide us with a placid, tractable patient. These drugs may be repeated in small increments during the operation, if necessary. It should be noted that the amount of diazepam and droperidol used is much lower than the usual recommended dosage.

PREMEDICATION ANTAGONISTS

We have used the same premedication routine for 20 years and have found it to be eminently satisfactory. However, the effects of any preanesthetic medication may be variable and, occasionally, paradoxical. Therefore, it is wise to have a standby program for using antagonists if one becomes concerned about respiratory depression, diminished response, or its antithesis, namely, hyperexcitability, restlessness, or dissociative phenomena.

Naloxone (Narcan) can be used as an antagonist of hydromorphone hydrochloride. Since it does not produce respiratory depression nor affect that produced by barbiturates, an absence of response to naloxone suggests that any depression is not due to the opiate. Its duration is short, so repeated doses may be necessary.

Physostigmine can be used to enhance the response to sensory stimulation, hasten arousal and the return of normal reflexes when these are impaired by pentobarbital. It reverses the central nervous system depression associated with diazepam and is the specific antagonist of scopolamine.

If one is operating in a same-day surgery or office facility, these antagonists can be used effectively to hasten recovery.

LOCAL ANESTHETIC AGENTS

Before infiltrating the nasal mucosa, we deaden it with cotton-tipped applicators that have been moistened with a mixture of 5% cocaine and 1:2000 epinephrine. This provides excellent, rapid surface anesthesia and produces intense vasoconstriction. We believe that the use of so-called cocaine mud is dangerous because one cannot be sure of the cocaine concentration, and it is well known that cocaine is readily absorbed after topical application, despite its vasoconstrictive properties.

Topical application of cocaine-moistened cotton pledgets to the gingivolabial sulcus of the upper lip in the premaxillary area will permit the base of the nose to be infiltrated with less pain. The maximum safe dose of 5% cocaine is said to be 4 ml (200 mg).

We use 6 to 8 ml of 1 or 2% lidocaine (Xylocaine) to obtain rapid, potent local infiltration anesthesia. Lidocaine has excellent powers of penetration and diffusion. It is usually combined with epinephrine to counteract its local vasodilating effect and to decrease the rate of systemic absorption so that its effectiveness is prolonged and larger doses of the agent can be used. The duration of anesthesia provided by the lidocaine is sufficiently long for most cosmetic facial operations.

The maximum safe dose of lidocaine with 1:100,000 epinephrine is 500 mg in 24 hours; this translates to 25 ml of 2% or 100 ml of 0.5%; if used without epinephrine, the maximum safe dose is 300 mg per 24 hours, that is, 15 ml of 2% or 60 ml of 0.5%.

GENERAL ANESTHESIA

Occasionally, a patient will demand a general anesthetic. Then, the anesthesiologist prescribes the premedication and selects the anesthetic agent to be used. However, we still infiltrate the nose with a local anesthetic containing epinephrine in an attempt to reduce intraoperative bleeding and the amount of the general anesthetic required.

Our experience has been that patients swell more and develop more ecchymosis when a general anesthetic is used, even though a local anesthetic containing epinephrine is used concomitantly.

LOCAL ANESTHETIC TECHNIQUE

The sensory innervation of the nose (Fig. 19) makes it ideal for local anesthesia, and we have used the following technique for many years.

1. The entire nasal mucosa is painted with cotton-tipped applicators, moistened with a solution consisting of equal parts of 10% cocaine and 1:1000 epinephrine.
2. Similarly moistened applicators are then placed over the sphenopalatine foramen and in the area where the anterior ethmoidal nerves enter the roof of each nasal cavity (Fig. 20). These are left in situ for about 5 minutes. This reduces the sensitivity of the nasal mucosa and makes subsequent injections of lidocaine more tolerable. It also produces intense vasoconstriction.
3. Using a 27 gauge needle on an offset syringe, we then inject the septal mucosa on each side with 2% lidocaine containing 1:100,000 epinephrine in three places: astride the course of the nasopalatine nerves, in the area of the internal nasal branches of the anterior ethmoidal nerves, and in the vicinity of the incisive canals (Fig. 21).
4. The undersurfaces of the bony pyramid are also injected to block the external nasal branches of the anterior ethmoidal nerves. This produces some anesthesia of the lobule and supratip areas (Fig. 22).
5. The anterior end of each inferior turbinate and adjacent tissue overlying the piriform margin are infiltrated. This partially deadens the lateral walls of the nasal vestibules supplied by infraorbital nerve branches, areas wherein incisions

will be made subsequently to permit lateral osteotomies (Fig. 23).

6. A small amount of anesthetic solution is injected into the supratip area (Fig. 24). After the region has become insensitive, the needle is advanced into four other areas to deposit anesthetic:
   a. Along the membranous septum down to the premaxilla (Fig. 25).
   b. Between the medial crura (Fig. 26).
   c. Along the entire length of each limen vestibula and extending as far as the nasofacial groove (Fig. 27).

7. The premaxillary floor of the nose is then infiltrated to block branches of the anterior superior alveolar nerves and some terminal branches of the infraorbital nerves. (Fig. 28).

8. Needles are then introduced through the midpoints of each limen vestibula (Fig. 29). The needles are kept as close to the skeleton as possible and are advanced along the middle of each lateral nasal wall until the sides of the radix nasi are reached. The solution is deposited as the needles are withdrawn to block the branches of the infratrochlear and infraorbital nerves supplying the lateral nasal walls. **Note:**It is not necessary to infiltrate the tissues overlying the nasofacial grooves because lidocaine can be "massaged" down into that area from the previous infiltration of the lateral nasal wall. This eliminates the possibility of perforating the angular vessels. It is unnecessary to inject anesthetic into the area of the infraorbital foramina thereby putting the infraorbital vessels at risk. Hematomas, thus produced before the actual operation starts, interfere with aesthetic accomplishments.

9. One half inch of roll gauze is then moistened with the topical anesthetic solution and inserted as loose packing into each nasal cavity (Fig. 30).

10. At least 10 minutes are allowed to elapse before the first incision is made.

We generally use about 6 ml of the cocaine-epinephrine mixture and from 6 to 8 ml of 2% lidocaine containing 1:100,000 epinephrine in the average rhinoplasty.

LOCAL ANESTHESIA CAVEATS

Before submitting any patient to an anesthetic regimen, his history should be thoroughly screened by the surgeon and a more extensive assessment made by the appropriate consultants, if necessary. Our self-administered history questionnaire (Fig. 2) has been helpful because of specific inquires of the patient's current and past medical history, the use of alcohol or recreational drugs, any untoward reactions to the drugs we normally use, and any medications currently being taken so that we might investigate possible incompatabilities with our routine.

Premedications and local anesthetics should be given sufficient time to act, the latter for at least 10 minutes. Too often we have seen patients taken to the operating room and have an operation started before their "on call" medications had a chance to reach full effectiveness; likewise, too many operations are started before the vasoconstrictor effect of the anesthetic solution becomes established.

Every person undergoing surgery should have an intravenous infusion started, a cardiac monitor connected. Resuscitative equipment and drugs should also be available.

The most dilute solution of the local anesthetic that is effective should be used, and the recommended dose should not be exceeded. Using a small caliber needle is helpful in preventing the use of too large a volume of solution.

Finally, the technique of local anesthetic injections can be artful, or it can be done crudely and with a heavy hand. Needles should be sharp and changed several times during the course of an infiltration, if necessary. They should not penetrate the skin at too acute an angle. One should be mindful of the location of large vessels so that they might be avoided. Injection should proceed in an orderly fashion from anesthetized to contiguous unanesthetized areas. Small amounts of solution should be injected with intermittent pressure as one proceeds, instead of rapidly and painfully expanding the tissues with large amounts.

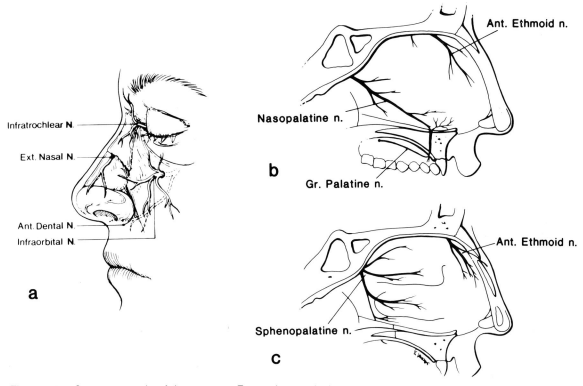

Figure 19.   Sensory supply of the nose. a: External nose. b: Nasal septum. c: Lateral wall of the internal nose.

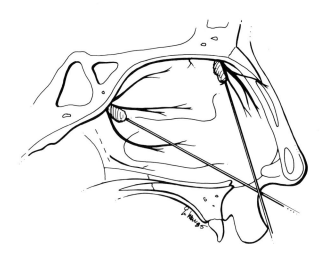

Figure 20.   Cotton-tipped applicators moistened with cocaine-epinephrine mixture placed in vicinity of sphenopalatine foramen and anterior ethmoidal nerves.

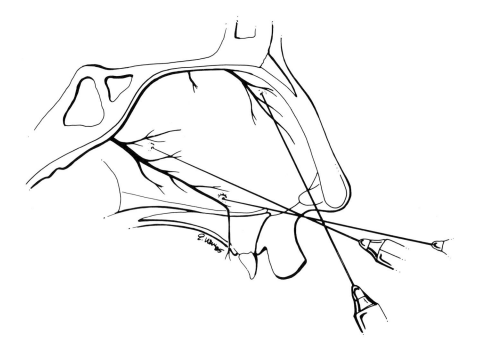

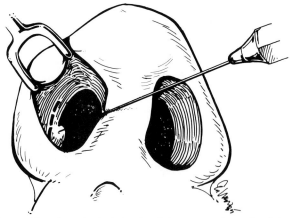

Figure 21. Injection of nasal septum with 2% lidocaine containing 1:100,000 epinephrine.

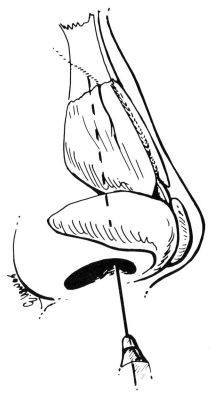

Figure 22. Injection of the undersurface of the bony pyramid to block the external branches of the anterior ethmoidal nerves that supply the lobule and supratip area.

Figure 23. Anesthetic injection into areas where the lateral osteotomies will be made later.

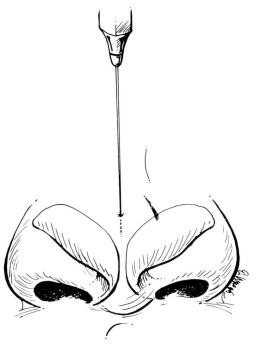

Figure 24. Anesthetic solution is injected into supratip area before injection into the surrounding areas.

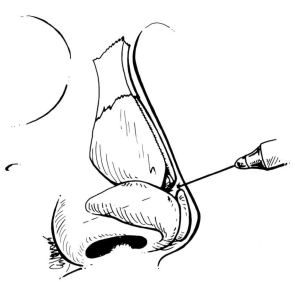

Figure 25. Needle is advanced down the membranous septum to the premaxillary area.

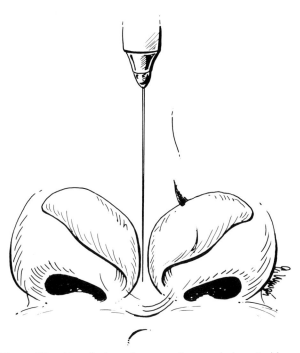

Figure 26. Needle from the supratip area is inserted between the medial crura.

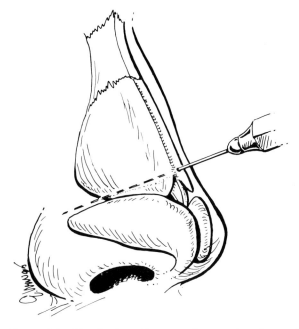

Figure 27. Needle from the supratip area is advanced along entire length of the limen vestibula to the nasofacial groove.

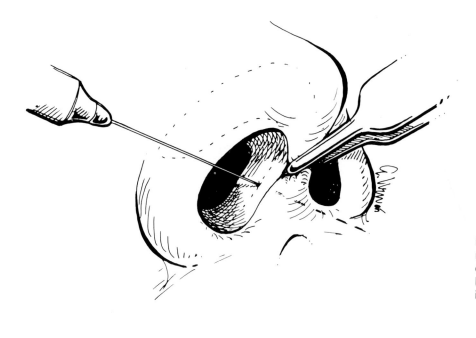

Figure 28. Injection of premaxillary area through previously anesthetized areas to block terminal branches of the infraorbital nerves.

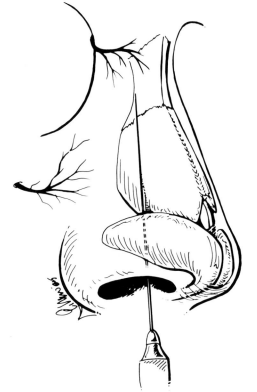

Figure 29. Anesthetization of the middle of the lateral nasal walls through the limen vestibula areas that were previously anesthetized.

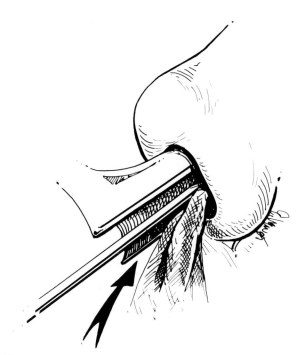

Figure 30. One-half inch roll gauze moistened with cocaine-epinephrine solution is packed loosely into each nasal cavity as the final step of the anesthetization procedure.

9   Overview of Technique

This short chapter provides an overview of the rhinoplasty technique currently used. We will discuss particulars of the various surgical steps in later chapters.

GENERAL CONSIDERATIONS

1. Local anesthesia is preferred in most instances.
2. Limen vestibula incisions are rarely used.
3. To minimize hemorrhage during surgery and unpredictable scar tissue and adhesion formation afterward, as much of the work as possible is done without cutting the nasal mucosa or the vestibular skin; the excess seems to contract during healing and has caused no trouble.
4. Nasal shortening is largely accomplished by modification of the lateral crura rather than by septal shortening.
5. Any septal straightening needed is performed at the same time as rhinoplasty; the procedures are never staged.
6. Osteotomies, the most traumatic part of rhinoplasty, are not done until the end of the operation. This reduces edema, which might otherwise interfere with the surgeon's judgment while attempting to make some of the more critical adjustments, for example, tip modification.

OPEN VERSUS CONVENTIONAL RHINOPLASTY

Several years ago, we became convinced of the value of open rhinoplasty and now use that approach more often than the conventional method. Endonasal rhinoplasty is virtually a blind procedure for the average surgeon. The open approach permits one to see more of the nasal skeleton, what is causing deformities, and the immediate effect of the corrective measures used; rhinoplasty therefore becomes a more precise and controllable procedure when done under direct vision.

Some surgeons fear the transcolumellar incision because of the possibility of unsightly scar formation. Our experience has been that the resultant scar becomes virtually imperceptible when the incision is properly located and meticulously closed; it has been said facetiously that only a person's dog might see it. However, patients are told in advance that the incision will be made but that the scar usually becomes almost invisible when it heals. Acceptance has been excellent; no one has ever balked after being told that the transcolumellar incision will permit better visualization for their surgeon. Incidentally, it has been puzzling to encounter resistance to transcolumellar incisions from the same surgeons who do not hesitate to use nearby external incisions to narrow widened alae.

Our experience has been that the open approach can be used to excellent advantage in any rhinoplasty. There are some instances, however, in which it is especially useful, for example, to repair combined deformities of the external nose and nasal septum, for the open reduction of old nasal fractures, for secondary rhinoplasty, particularly when excessive soft tissue in the supratip area is a problem, for deformities accompanying cleft lip and palates, when the alar cartilages are remarkably enlarged or distorted, and when it becomes necessary to lengthen the nasal dorsum.

ORDER OF OPERATION

I.   Exposure
     A.   Conventional rhinoplasty
         1.   Transfixion incision may or may not be used
         2.   Bilateral cartilage-splitting incisions are made through the lateral crura parallel to and 3 to 5 mm below the limen vestibula
         3.   Transfixion and cartilage-splitting incisions are connected
         4.   After the scrolls of the lateral crura

have been excised, the soft tissues overlying the upper lateral cartilages and the dorsum of the cartilagenous septum are elevated

B. Open rhinoplasty (Fig. 31)

1. A transverse incision is made through the skin of the columella several millimeters above the flared free ends of the medial crura

2. Incisions are then made along the caudal ends of each medial crus; they extend from the level of the nostril apices to the lateral ends of the transcolumellar skin incision

3. The columellar skin overlying the medial crus is elevated by blunt dissection

4. Incisions are then made along the entire length of the caudal margin of each lateral crus and connected to the medial crural incisions

5. The tissues overlying the alar cartilages and the entire upper cartilagenous vault are elevated

C. In both conventional and open rhinoplasty, the periosteum over the medial portions of the nasal bones is elevated in preparation for hump removal (Fig. 32)

II. Lower lateral cartilage modification

A. Conventional rhinoplasty

1. May be accomplished by the retrograde method, by the eversion method, or by the delivery technique

2. Medial-lateral crura continuity may or may not be interrupted at the angle; the lateral crura may be transected laterally. Vestibular skin need not be cut if the delivery or retrograde technique are used; otherwise, it must be cut along with the cartilage

B. Open rhinoplasty. Since the entire lower cartilagenous area is exposed, any incisions or excisions may be made without cutting the underlying vestibular skin

III. Mucosal tunnels are created beneath the junction of the upper lateral cartilages and the nasal septum to permit intramucosal hump removal later. In conventional rhinoplasty, mucosal elevation is begun at the upper end of the transfixion incision; in open rhinoplasty, the domes of alar cartilage are separated, the septal angle exposed, and elevation of the mucosa begins in this area

IV. Upper lateral cartilages are cut from the septum intramucosally

V. Some of the excess projection of the cartilagenous septal dorsum is excised beginning at the rhinion; this makes the rhinion prominent

VI. Nasal hump is removed intramucosally

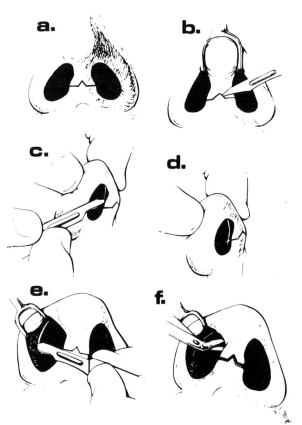

Figure 31. a and b: Transcolumellar incision; the center of the incision is best made with a no. 11 knife blade. c: Incisions are next made along the caudal ends of the medial crura. d: Incisions are joined and tissues scored beyond the ends of each to form an "X" that facilitates accurate approximation later during closure. e: Incisions made along caudal ends of lateral crura. f: Undermining proceeds with angulated Converse scissors.

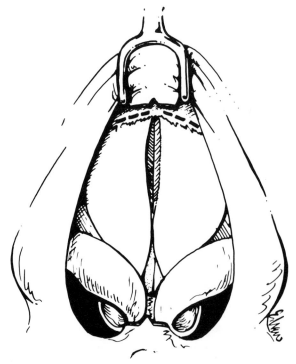

Figure 32. Incisions are made through the periosteum about 1 mm above the caudal ends of the nasal bones to permit periosteal elevation before hump removal.

VII. A submucous resection or septoplasty is performed if indicated; the caudal end of the septum is splinted when dislocated cartilage is shifted to the midline

VIII. Medial and lateral osteotomies are performed to permit nasal pyramid narrowing

IX. Final adjustments are made to the nasal bones, the cartilagenous dorsum, the upper lateral cartilages and the tip cartilage

X. The incisions are sutured

XI. Alar width is lessened if necessary

XII. An external dressing is applied

10　Incisions and Skeletal Exposure

INCISIONS

A variety of incisions may be used to expose the skeletal structures of the nose and to undermine the overlying soft tissues so that they might readjust to the remodeled contour after operation. The most common ones are: the transfixion incision, limen vestibula incisions, several types of cartilage-splitting incisions, marginal incisions made along the caudal edges of the alar cartilages, a transcolumellar skin incision for open rhinoplasty, and incisions to permit lateral osteotomies.

Incisions made to separate the upper lateral cartilages from the dorsum of the septal cartilage will not be discussed because they are performed intramucosally.

Transfixion Incision

The purpose of this incision through the membranous septum (Fig. 33) is to provide access to the caudal end of the septal cartilage and the nasal spine; sometimes it is used for columellar advancement when increased tip projection is desired. The incision follows the cephalic margins of the medial crura. It extends downward from the apices of the internal soft triangles located at the upper end of the membranous septum and terminates just short of the flared ends of the medial crura. Sometimes it is extended to the level of the nostril floor when tip projection is to be increased.

Generally, the transfixion incision is described as being made after elevation of the tissues overlying the cartilagenous vault of the nose, in fact, as an extension of that maneuver. On two occasions we have seen inexperienced operators cut through the columella when attempting to do this; therefore, we suggest that the transfixion incision be made first to eliminate that danger.

The incision closely follows the cephalic margins of the medial crura instead of the caudal end of the septal cartilage, which lessens possible adverse effects of scarring in the membranous septum when adjacent cartilage is excised. Better scars have resulted from incising near the medial crura.

Stopping the transfixion incision above the flared lower ends of the medial crura instead of "completing" it, as was previously taught, preserves the base of the columella for later use. For example, a pocket into which implants can be introduced can be created there, if necessary. In addition, the area below the medial crura has no cartilage skeleton to forestall unfavorable scar contracture. Finally, it avoids damage to the fat pad found at the base of the columella in young people; atrophy of this tissue can lead to a loss of tip projection. Cutting short the incision still leaves sufficient working room to permit removal of subcutaneous tissue when narrowing the columellar base, to modify the nasal spine, or to sever the depressor septi muscle, if necessary. Actually, the length of the transfixion may be varied by ending it anywhere along the membranous septum. It is even possible to perform rhinoplasty without a transfixion incision if no work on the caudal septum or the nasal spine is intended.

Some surgeons use what is known as a "hemitransfixion," an incision made through one side of the membranous septum only. This eliminates one incision, but the surgical balance and better exposure that bilateral incisions provide would seem preferable, particularly when dealing with a distorted caudal septum and columella.

Limen Vestibula Incisions

Limen vestibula incisions provide access to the nasal dorsum. When combined with the transfixion incision, they separate most of the alar complex from the remainder of the nasal skeleton.

The cuts should be located between the upper and lower lateral cartilages. Often, they are inadvertently made through the lateral crura scrolls, thereby leaving part of those structures attached to the caudal ends of the upper lateral cartilages. Unless removed, these remnants of the scrolls will cause postoperative thickening, or lumpiness, in the lateral infratip lobule area.

The incisions are begun medially as a continuation of the transfixion incision. They are extended lateralward along the entire length of the body of each lateral crus (Fig. 34a).

We rarely use limen vestibula incisions because cartilage-splitting incisions offer more advantages, including better visibility.

Cartilage-Splitting Incisions

These incisions are made through both the vestibular skin and underlying lateral crura. They are usually located from 3 to 5 mm caudal to the limen vestibula, the distance depending on how great a modification of the alar complex is planned. They run parallel to the limen and extend from the upper ends of the transfixion incision to the lateral end of each lateral crus (Fig. 34b).

Thus, the lateral crura are divided into two parts: small upper segments, consisting of little more than the scrolls, and wider lower segments comprising the remainder of the crura.

The cartilage of the upper segments is dissected free from its attachments and removed. This provides access to the remainder of the cartilagenous skeleton so that a plane of dissection can be made continuous with the transfixion incision.

The excellence of these incisions stems from the fact that, unlike limen vestibula incisions, they are located some distance away from the nasal valve area so those important structures are less likely to be periled by scar tissue contracture during healing. In this connection, they help to reduce significantly the number of intranasal incisions when used with the intramucosal technique, especially when minimal alar cartilage modification is required. To elucidate: if after limen vestibula and transfixion incisions the upper lateral cartilages are cut from the septum and shortened, there will be a confluence of eight incisions in the valve area; two more will be added, for a total of ten, if vertical incisions are made through the angles of the alar cartilages for tip modification (Fig. 35). Since no one can yet predict how capricious scar contracture will be, it should be apparent that aesthetic and functional results may be jeopardized. No other situation in plastic surgery comes to mind where good results are expected when so many incisions have a common meeting point; it seems sufficient to note that stellate scars are usually not good scars.

There are other benefits. Enough alar cartilage remains so that any of the usual technique of tip modification can be used subsequently. Also, the possibility of leaving part of the scrolls behind is lessened.

Other type of cartilage-splitting incisions are used in the nasal vestibule, but they are not specifically designed to provide access to the cartilagenous skeleton (Fig. 36). For example, they may be used to divide the alar cartilages at their angles or domes or to transect the lateral parts of the lateral crura. In effect, they are done to effect lobule modification and rotation or to alter tip projection.

Marginal Incisions

Marginal incisions follow the caudal margins of the alar cartilages (Fig. 37). They may be made either with a scalpel or with iris scissors. In either case, a studied effort should be made to keep close to the cartilages; otherwise, their edges may be nicked, or tenting of the skin over the soft tissue triangles may occur postoperatively due to scar tissue contracture.

The length of the marginal incisions depends on how the alar cartilages are to be treated. If each lateral crus is to be converted into a pedicled chondroplastic flap for delivery through the nostril, the incision will be extended lateralward from the apices of the respective soft triangles as far as is necessary to provide sufficient exposure. On the other hand, if the alar cartilages are to be converted into bipedicled chondroplastic flaps in preparation for delivery, the incisions must, also, be extended for varying distances along the caudal ends of the medial crura.

The main use of marginal incisions is to permit modification of the alar cartilages, but they can also be used to provide access to the cartilagenous dorsum and to the caudal end of the septum.

Transcolumellar Incision

The transcolumellar incision is used in open rhinoplasty (Fig. 38). It is made through the skin of the columella and stops just short of the flared free ends of the medial crura. It should not be positioned below that level because there is no cartilage skeleton to resist tensions generated during healing.

The center of the incision is triangulated to improve the appearance of the subsequent scar and to provide three landmarks for accurate closure; it is best made with a no. 11 surgical blade. The remainder is made a with no. 15 blade and joins the inferior ends of marginal incisions caudal to the medial crura.

Lateral Osteotomy Incisions

Incisions to permit introduction of instruments for performance of lateral osteotomy are made over the rims of the piriform opening. They are located immediately cephalic to the attachment of the anterior ends of the inferior nasal turbinates and are directed parallel to the bony rim (Fig. 39). They are usually made about 10 mm long with a no. 11 blade. The blade is swept for a short distance on both sides of the bone to cut the attached tissue therefrom. Then, a short perpendicuarly directed incision is made through the underlying periosteum to facilitate creation of subperiosteal tunnels to accommodate the instruments.

EXPOSURE OF SKELETAL ELEMENTS

Once access incisions have been made, the elevation of soft tissue from the skeletal dorsum can proceed. This is done by a combination of sharp and blunt dissection with a fine point iris scissors.

It is important to keep the plane of dissection as close to the skeleton as possible, below the level of most of the blood vessels of the external nose and below the level of the nasal muscles. This reduces bleeding and postoperative reaction. Of equal importance is the extent of the undermining. Over the cartilagenous vault, it should extend to the piriform margins in all directions to assure maximum drapeage of the skin over the skeletal contour postoperatively (Fig. 40).

When the nasal bones are reached, the periosteum is incised 1 mm above and parallel to their caudal margins (Fig. 41). It is then elevated as far as the nasofrontal suture line so that the nasal hump can be removed subperiosteally and the medial osteotomy will not lacerate it. We try to preserve as much periosteum as possible because we believe it acts to minimize any roughness of the dorsum resulting from hump removal or narrowing of the nasal pyramid. Also, it serves as a barrier between the subcutaneous tissue and nasal mucosa, thereby eliminating the possibility of them becoming attached to each other during healing and causing dimpling of the overlying skin.

In open rhinoplasty, the skin above the transcolumellar incision is elevated from the caudal margins or the medial crura, from the dome and bodies of the lateral crura, and from at least part of their lateral extensions (Fig. 42). The extent of tissue elevation from the lateral crura is the same as when those structures are delivered through the nostrils as unilateral or bilateral chondroplastic flaps.

The septal cartilage may be exposed by splitting the membranous septum after transfixion or by cutting the upper lateral cartilages from the septal dorsum with a scalpel or sharp scissors and then elevating the underlying septal mucosa (Figs. 43,44).

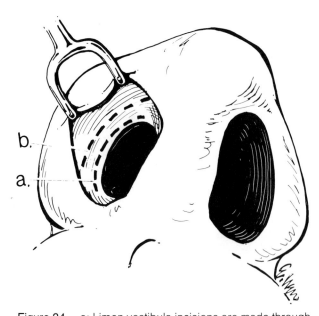

Figure 33. The transfixion incision. We recommend that it be made along the cephalic margins of the medial crura for reasons cited in the text. It extends from the apices of the internal soft triangles to just short of the flared ends of the medial crura inferiorly.

Figure 34. a: Limen vestibula incisions are made through the vestibular skin between the upper and lower lateral cartilages; they are continuous with the upper ends of the transfixion incision. b: Cartilage-splitting incisions are made parallel to the limen vestibula and through the vestibular skin and lateral crura. The distance from the limen depends on how much excision of the lateral crura is desired.

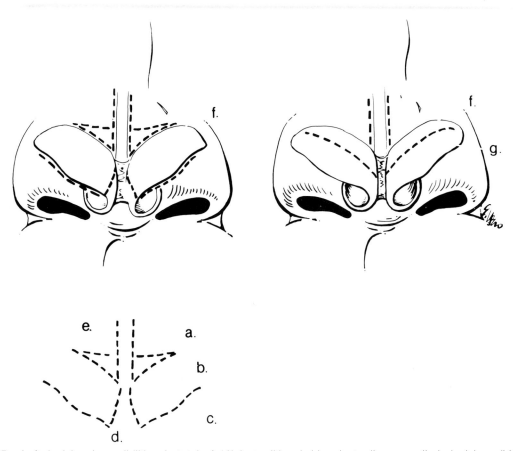

Figure 35. Left: Incisional possibilities (a total of 12) in traditional rhinoplasty: limen vestibula incisions (b), marginal incisions (c), angle or dome incisions (d), incisions cutting upper lateral cartilages from the septum (e), location of the upper end of the transfixions incision (f), incisions made to shorten upper lateral cartilages (a). Right: When cartilage-splitting incisions and the intramucosal technique are used, only four incisions are needed: bilateral cartilage-splitting incisions (g) that are continuous with the transfixion incision (f).

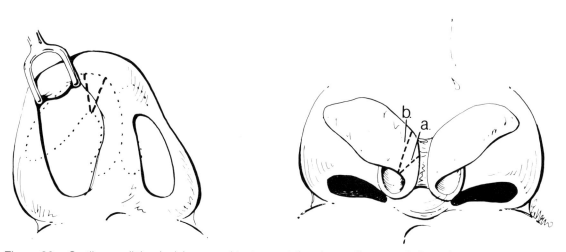

Figure 36. Cartilage-splitting incisions used to transect the alar cartilages at their angles (a) or at their domes.

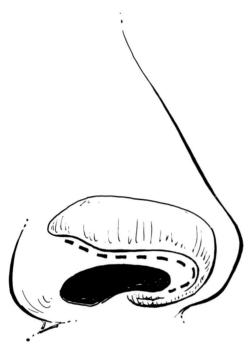

Figure 37. Marginal incisions follow the caudal margin of the alar cartilage to permit surgical exposure of those structures.

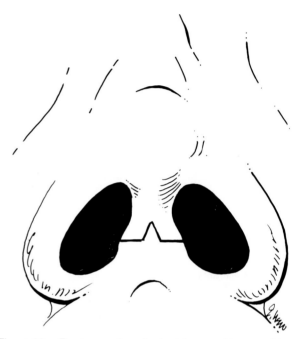

Figure 38. The transcolumellar incision used in open rhinoplasty is made just above the flared lower ends of the medial crura.

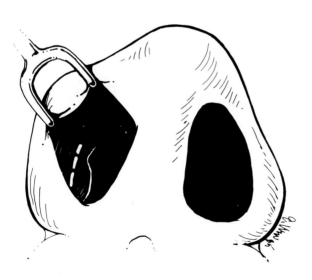

Figure 39. The incisions for lateral osteotomy are made through vestibular skin near the anterior ends of the inferior turbinates. They are directed parallel to the piriform margin.

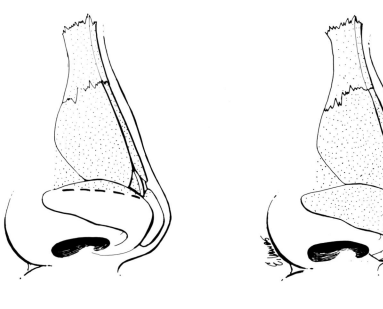

Figure 40. Amount of skin and subcutaneous tissue undermining in rhinoplasty. Left: In the average conventional operation. Right: When open rhinoplasty is performed.

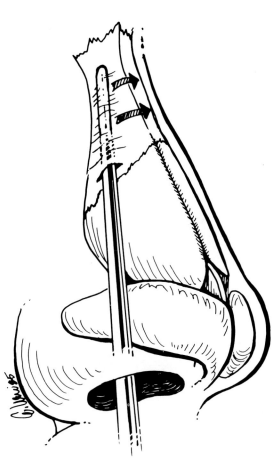

Figure 41. Periosteal elevation before hump removal.

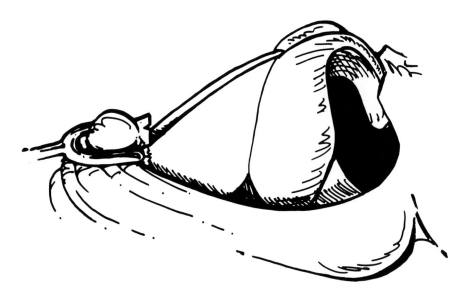

Figure 42. Skin elevation and skeletal exposure possible with the open rhinoplasty technique.

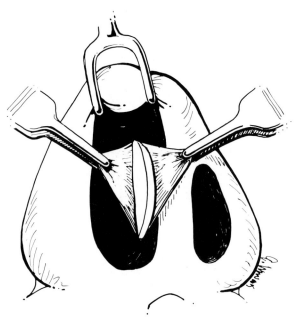

Figure 43. Exposure of the caudal end of the septum through a transfixion incision.

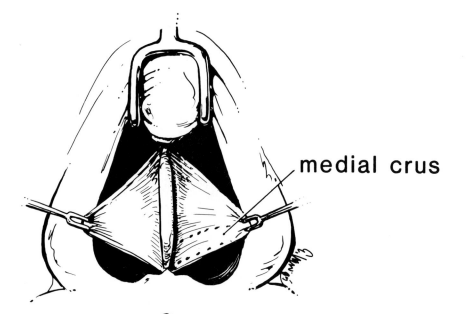

medial crus

Figure 44. Exposure of the caudal end of the septal cartilage via the external rhinoplasty approach. The medial crura above the transcolumellar incision are separated, as are the leaves of the membranous septum.

11 Surgery of the Nasal Base: Setting Tip Projection and Location

Nasal base surgery consists of more than remodeling the lobule; it also plays an important part in shortening the nose as well as in determining how much hump removal is necessary.

Pressing the columella against the caudal septum will reveal that most noses are too long because of the length, width, and direction of the lateral crura (Fig. 45); that is why it is rarely necessary to trim the caudal septum, as was formerly taught (Fig. 46). Sufficient shortening can usually be achieved by merely modifying the lateral crura. In fact, what is done to remodel the lobule often helps to shorten the nose.

Once the nose has been shortened by rotating the base cephalward, the projection of the tip in its new location dictates how much hump should be removed. Fortunately, the surgeon can control tip projection to a large extent; it can be increased, decreased, or left alone as aesthetic canons require.

Secondary aims of nasal base surgery include the correction of columellar abnormalities and distortions of the alae and nostrils. To recapitulate, the aims of nasal base surgery are:

1. To remodel the lobule
2. To rotate the tip cephalward (to shorten the nose)
3. To increase, decrease, or maintain the tip's projection in its new location
4. To correct columellar abnormalities
5. To correct nostril and alar distortions

TERMINOLOGY

The dynamics of nasal base surgery are difficult to understand and the relationships of the basal cartilages are complex, but the problem has been compounded by muddled terminology. Thus, a review of Chapter 6 is recommended; even so, it would seem worthwhile to spotlight some of the terms (Fig. 47):

1. The nasal base: The area of the nose formed by the conjoined lower lateral cartilage; often erroneously referred to as the nasal tip
2. The tip of the nose: The free angle formed by the rounding of the medial and lateral crura
3. The lobule: That part of the base located above the level of the upper rims of the nostrils
4. The infratip lobule: The portion of the lobule located between the nasal tip and the nostrils
5. The soft tissue triangles: The soft tissue spanning the fissure between the medial and lateral crura; the external triangles bridge the caudal margins of the crura and are often visible on the caudal aspect of the infratip lobule, whereas the internal ones are located between the cephalic margins, at the upper ends of the membranous septum
6. The angles versus the domes of the lower lateral cartilages: The angle is the narrow portion, genu or isthmus, that marks the junction of the lateral and medial crus; it can be located by drawing an imaginary line between the apexes of the external and internal soft tissue triangles. On the other hand, the dome is the highest part of the nasal vestibule; it represents the highest part of the concavity formed by the inner surface of the lateral crus and is composed mostly of lateral crus. The further the domes are from the midline, the wider, and, usually, flatter, will the lobule be (Fig. 48).
7. The hinge of the lateral crus: The flexible area between the body of the cartilage and its accessory cartilages or its lateral continuation along the piriform margin (Fig. 49); it bends inward when

the base of the nose is rotated in a cephalic direction

8. The scroll: The curved cephalic margin of the lateral crus that overlies the adjacent upper lateral cartilage. It becomes juxtaposed to the scroll of the opposite lateral crus as it proceeds medially; sometimes, it extends into the medial crus

9. The nostril sill: The continuation of the alar margins toward the base of the columella

10. Tip projection: The distance from the facial plane to the tip of the lobule

11. Lobular definition: A state wherein the planes and angles of the lobule are sculptured sufficiently to make the structure distinct rather than amorphous looking.

TRIPOD ANALOGY: SURGICAL APPLICATIONS

The conjoined lower lateral cartilages bear a striking resemblance to a tilted tripod attached to the caudal end of the nose; the structure is tilted because one leg is formed by the united medial crura whose length is always shorter than the lateral crura that form the other two legs (Fig. 50).

Thinking in terms of tripod modification allows one to employ mechanical principles to rotate the nasal base and alter tip projection. The nose can be shortened by shortening the longer legs of the tripod (the lateral crura) in some manner and, if necessary, by modifying the caudal end of the septal cartilage to increase the amplitude of medial crura rotation. To increase tip projection, the shorter leg of the tripod (the united medial crura) would have to be lengthened. If decreased projection of the tip is desired, both the short and long legs of the tripod are reduced in length (Fig. 51).

To be sure, there are other factors that influence the execution of these principles; for example, the length, width, and direction of the lateral crura, the inherent curvatures of the alar cartilages, the caudal ends of the upper lateral cartilages, the quality and elasticity of the overlying skin and soft tissues, the length of the nasal septum, the width of the medial crura, and disharmony between the levels of the medial and lateral crura.

The tripod has several supports or attachments to the rest of the nose (Fig 52). It is important to know about them because some or all may be weakened during rhinoplasty, and failure to compensate for the weakening can adversely affect the operative results. The supports include:

1. A soft tissue sling that connects the medial ends of the lateral crura and spans the caudal end of the septum; it has been termed a "ligament." This support can be compromised or destroyed in a number of ways: when the projection of the septal dorsum is reduced, even though the ligament remains intact; when the lateral crura are separated, as during delivery through the nostrils for modification; when the medial ends of the scrolls or the ends of the lateral crura are excised during lobule remodeling; when the alar cartilages are separated during open rhinoplasty to gain access to the caudal septum and the nasal spine.

2. A similar sling of tissue joins the medial crura; it is particularly important where the lower ends of the medial crura overlap the caudal end of the septum in a tongue-in-groove arrangement. Excision of septal cartilage in the area of overlap will cause dramatic settling of the tripod in the direction of the premaxilla.

3. The scrolls of the lateral crura overlap the caudal ends of the upper lateral cartilages and are joined to them by fibrous tissue that is divided by limen vestibula incisions and destroyed by excision of alar cartilage from the area.

4. The length of the medial crura determines how much the tripod can settle if other supports, for example, the medial crura-caudal septum overlap, are weakened. Their length varies (Fig. 53); if they are too short, they may have to be shored up to prevent excessive settling after operation.

5. The membranous septum has some small supportive function, especially if the other major supports have been damaged.

6. The premaxillary accumulation of fat. If it atrophies as a result of surgical trauma or aging, the tripod will settle, the extent depending on the length of the medial crura and the strength of the medial crura-septum overlap. This is one explanation for the insidious development of nasal humps as people age.

7. The lateral crura also support the tripod

as a result of their rigidity and attachment to the upper lateral cartilages.

There is no doubt that the three major supports of the basal skeleton are the septal dorsum, the medial crura-septum overlap, and the medial crura themselves. Proof is evident when the caudal end of the septum is destroyed by infection or trauma: the tripod settles to the face as much as the length of the medial crura will permit.

DYNAMICS OF NASAL BASE ROTATION

When the tripod is rotated upward, each lateral crus will bow outward; unless shortened to eliminate the bow, they will push the tip of the nose downward postoperatively (that is, the tip will drop or "droop"). This causes the soft tissue in the supratip area to thicken and produces a rounding of the area known as a "soft tissue polly beak deformity" (Fig. 54).

The crura can be shortened in two ways (Fig. 55). First, by removing a segment of cartilage from the hinge areas, the amount depending on how much cartilage overlap occurs after the cartilages are transected. The shape of the excised segments will be determined by the amount of nasal base rotation and the amount of tip projection desired after rotation has been accomplished; it may be triangular, rectangular, or trapezoidal. Second, by dividing the alar cartilages at their angles. This permits the medial crura to be rotated independently of the lateral crura, their rotation being limited by the caudal end of the nasal septum. The medial ends of the lateral crura will usually overlap the upper ends of the medial crura when the alar cartilages are divided at their angles; the areas of overlap are then excised. This second method is particularly applicable when only small amounts of nasal base rotation are needed; one of its virtues is that it facilitates lobule remodeling. The two methods of shortening are often combined.

Shortening the lateral crura is not the only factor involved in tripod rotation:

1. The scrolls of the lateral crura must be excised usually; excisions extended to the hinge area will facilitate rotation of the crura but will not shorten them; they will still bow unless segments of cartilage are removed.

2. The skin overlying the cartilagenous dorsum is important. It must be elastic enough to permit rotation; otherwise

the nasal tip will droop postoperatively. Skin pliability can be improved by removal of excess subcutaneous tissue and crosshatching the under surface of the dermis.

3. The caudal ends of the upper lateral cartilages may have to be excised because they are too long or because they curve upward ("returning"). Although they may cause lobule widening, they do not contribute to the length of the nose per se (Fig. 56).

4. The caudal septum should be trimmed only when surgery on the lateral crura fails to achieve the desired amount of nasal base rotation.

DYNAMICS OF TIP PROJECTION

The game plan in rhinoplasty may require that tip projection be increased, decreased, or maintained. Decreasing or maintaining projection is not difficult, but increasing it is.

Of primary importance is the length of the medial crura; they may fill any part or all of the columella (Fig. 53). Their length determines what will happen if the tripod supports are weakened or destroyed. Projection will not decrease if they extend the whole length of the columella; otherwise, it will decrease until the lower ends of the crura can descend no more, that is, when they reach the level of the floor of the nasal vestibule.

To maintain tip projection, one should try not to disrupt the medial crura-septum overlap; when it becomes necessary to do so, the joint should be reestablished at the end of the operation and stabilized for a few weeks with a strong synthetic septocolumellar suture until healing occurs. When it becomes necessary to excise part of the caudal septum, the medial crura may be lengthened with a shoring strut of septal cartilage that is inserted either between or caudal to the crura; cartilage for this purpose is obtained from the patient's own septum or from a cartilage bank. The strut extends upward from a point about 2 mm above the premaxillary crest to as high as the level of the nostril apexes (Fig. 57).

Tip projection can be decreased by destroying the supports of the tripod or by shortening its legs. The main supports (Fig. 52) are destroyed by interrupting the "ligaments" connecting the medial ends of the lateral crura, by lowering the projection of the septal dorsum, and by excising cartilage from the region of the inferior septal angle. The lateral and medial legs of the tripod can be shortened by excising cartilage. We have decreased projection by as much as 10 mm by using a combination of these measures.

Tip projection can be increased in several ways (Fig. 58). Narrowing a widened columella base helps. Any excess intracrural soft tissue should be excised, and it may be necessary to transect the lower ends of both medial crura; then, the columella base is "gathered" with a nonabsorbable septocolumellar suture for at least 3 weeks.

Onlay grafts of morselized cartilage placed atop intact domes will help also; before their placement, however, the upper ends of the medial crura should be strengthened by sewing them together; likewise, any domal vestibular skin that remains after excision of the scrolls should be sewn together over the caudal end of the septal dorsum to eliminate a potential dead space in the supratip area and to help maintain projection of the tip above the level of the septal dorsum.

The convexity of the lateral crura that remains after the scrolls have been removed can be used to advantage. Flattening the convexity will lengthen the crura, which can then be used to increase tip projection. The flattening is best accomplished by transecting the alar cartilages at their angles and dissecting the vestibular skin away from the undersurfaces of the lateral crura. The increased tip projection this affords will not be maintained unless the upper ends of the medial crura are lengthened to frustrate the effects of healing that would ordinarily cause the ends of the lateral crura to bend downward again. In practice, morselized onlay grafts are positioned above the sutured ends of the medial crura and beneath the medial ends of the lateral crura.

Two things should be noted. First, any increase of tip projection achieved by modifying the tripod apex in the manner just described will also increase the height of the lobule and could upset the columella to lobule ratio if carried too far. This is one of the dangers of dividing the alar cartilages too far lateral to their angles and sewing them together to elongate the short leg of the tripod (Fig. 57). The second concerns the use of so-called shield grafts, an old procedure recently resurrected by Sheen; they add little to tip projection; rather, they modify the infratip lobule but improve the appearance of the entire structure.

Struts fashioned from septal cartilage can be inserted between the medial crura to increase their length and improve tip projection. However, a word of caution is in order. Cartilage implants absorb if subjected to too much tension, so the surrounding tissues of the upper lip and premaxillae must be widely undermined, shifted medialward, and, then, immobilized with a strong nonabsorbable suture for several weeks. A lesser procedure that is sometimes appropriate consists of removing a rectangular section from the caudal septum to create more room for the columella to move. Finally, whenever cartilage struts are used, they should be made to stop short of reaching the premaxillary crest; otherwise, they will veer from the midline and cause columellar deviation.

In addition to using intercrural columellar struts, the premaxillary area just below the nasal spine can be augmented with cartilage or with a synthetic material (such as a roll of Supramid mesh); they are inserted through an opening created by separating the medial crura and dissecting away tissues attached to the nasal spine, piriform margins, and premaxillae.

LOBULE MODIFICATION

The aim of lobular surgery is to cause the structure to resemble an equilateral triangle when viewed from below and to fill no more than two-thirds of the intercanthal distance when viewed from the front. Additionally, correction of various asymmetries may be required. The method of increasing lobular height was described when methods of increasing tip projection were considered.

To narrow the lobule, the domes must be moved closer to the angles of the alar cartilages and varying amounts of the scrolls must be excised; if the scrolls extend into the upper ends of the medial crura, excision should extend into that area, too. Scroll excision changes the inherent structural tensions at the tips of the alar cartilages, but this is of little import if the lobule is only slightly widened beforehand or if the upper ends of the medial crura were not distorted, as is frequently the case (Fig. 59). The cartilages need not be divided at their angles in such instances; otherwise, they should be separated so that the tensions can be dissipated, if not, unsightly knoblike protuberances called bosses and other asymmetries will develop postoperatively (Fig. 60).

When the lateral crura overlap the upper ends of the medial crura, the surplus cartilage is excised, an attempt being made to reproduce nature as far as possible; each is trimmed to articulate with two structures, the ipsilateral medial crus and the cephalic border of the opposite lateral crus.

The following should be considered.

1. The upper ends of the medial crura are important in narrowing the lobule; they should not be sewn together until they are narrowed by excision of an appropriate amount of their cephalic borders.
2. Lobular asymmetries may require excision of unequal amounts of cartilage

or the introduction of appropriately trimmed cartilage implants.

3. Concavities of the lateral crura are best handled by, first, determining how much can be improved by excisions from their cephalic borders and, then, by using wafers of morselized cartilage to obliterate any of the depression remaining. Convexities may be corrected by thinning the cartilage with a scapel or by morselization.

4. Marked crookedness of the medial crura can be corrected by excising strips of cartilage from the bends and, then, suturing the remainder to a solid intercrural strut of cartilage.

NOSTRIL NARROWING

Nostril narrowing during rhinoplasty deserves more attention than it gets; some surgeons claim that they never narrow the nostrils, a practice that seems inconsistent with what we know about the dynamics of the operation. Nostrils that are wide preoperatively certainly should be narrowed because they will be too wide after operation.

Sometimes, wideness is produced by the operation. When the supports of the tripod are weakened, the short leg sinks toward the face and the alae bow outward, usually causing a change in the direction of the long axes of the nostrils. Additionally, rotation of the base causes more of the nostrils to become visible, so any flaring that exists will be more noticeable; in fact, on occasion, we have modified the nostril bases for aesthetic reasons even though the alae did not extend beyond the intercanthal boundries.

The technique selected depends on the configuration of the alae, whether they are continuous with a well-defined nostril sill or are attached directly to the face. Finally, the width of the base of the columella is a consideration because, at times, narrowing of that area changes the type of modification that is selected, or it may eliminate the need for the procedure. Parenthetically, nostril surgery should never be done before the remainder of the operation has been completed.

The method we usually use consists of excision of wedges from the sills and conversion of the alae into rotation-advancement flaps by using backcuts. The design of the wedges is dictated by the problem at hand; in general, they are triangular or rectangular (Fig. 61).

The incisions are made with a no. 11 blade whose cutting edge is directed upward into the nostril. The lateral cut is made first; it starts as a stab incision begun 1 or 2 mm above the alar-facial groove and is completed with sawlike movements of the blade. After the medial cuts have been made, the two incisons are connected to permit removal of the wedge. Then 5 to 6 mm backcuts are made into the alae to permit their rotation; shorter cuts may be made in the direction of the columella base. If there is an accessory sill on the inner surface of the alae, it is corrected by excising a triangular wedge whose base extends medially into the original wound.

The method and sequence of suturing is important, otherwise closure will suffer. After bleeding is controlled with bipolar cautery, the nostril margin is carefully aligned, and the first 4-0 polypropylene suture is introduced through the whole thickness of the epithelium. The remainder of the external sutures is inserted before internal suturing is started. The true effectiveness of the procedure on nostril contour cannot be appreciated until all suturing has been finished.

The external sutures are removed in 3 days, and the wound is reinforced with Steri-Strips for an additional 4 days, at which time the inner sutures are taken out. The resulting scars are usually minimal and represent an acceptable trade-off, in our opinion.

As simple as this procedure is surgically, some caveats are in order:

1. If a surgeon wonders, even fleetingly, whether he should do wedge resections when completing a rhinoplasty, he should probably go ahead and do them; it is better to do them at the time of operation than as a separate procedure later.

2. Wedge resections can cause slight distortion of the upper reaches of the alae and the nostril apexes if the alar cartilages have not been divided at their angles. This does not preclude their use in such instances if they are necessary, however.

3. A small amount of nostril margin curvature that exists where the alae join the sills should be preserved when making the lateral incision; this will avert distortion of the nostril contour caused by subsequent closure of the incisions (Fig. 62).

4. The medial incisions should not violate the columellar base.

5. Backcuts into the alae should always be located 1 or 2 mm above the alar-facial grooves; placement in the grooves frequently causes irregular healing, scarring, and other problems.

When the alae join the face directly instead of continuing into the nostril sills, correction is not so neat in that the resultant scars have higher visibility. Narrowing is accomplished by excising tissue from the nostril floor or by performing Z-plasties to move the alae medially.

OPERATIVE STEPS

It is difficult to describe nasal base surgery in cookbook fashion because of its complexity; it is best learned piecemeal at surgical demonstrations.

The external rhinoplasty approach has made surgery easier and more precise because it permits the surgeon to modify the alar cartilages under direct vision, and the correction can be accomplished without violating the integrity of the underlying vestibular skin.

1. The domes are separated down to the level of the septal dorsum, or further if wider exposure is needed to work on the caudal septum, the nasal spine, or in the premaxillary area; any remnants of soft tissue are removed. These maneuvers result in a slight increase of tip projection (Fig. 63).

2. Equal amounts of cartilage are excised from the cephalic borders of each lateral crus, beginning at the level of the septal dorsum and extending to the hinge areas. The excisions are then extended over the domes to end at the angles. If the scrolls continue into the upper ends of the medial crura, they are removed from that area, too. Several changes result from these excisions: the tip becomes narrower, its projection increases slightly, and the lateral crura left behind consist of strips of cartilage that are 5 to 6 mm wide at their widest points (Fig. 64).

3. If more tip narrowing is desired, the alar cartilages are transected at their angles and the vestibular epithelium dissected from the adjacent ends of both crura (medial and lateral) for a short distance so they become straighter (Fig. 65). Excising the cephalic borders of the upper ends of the medial crura will narrow the tip even more.

4. When a columella strut is required for tip support, a tunnel between the medial crura is prepared to receive it. Ordinarily, little more is needed than creating the opening with straight iris scissors.

However, when the medial crura have been separated along their entire length and the base of the columella and premaxillary area have been opened, the entire area must be closed with mattress sutures of 4–0 polyglactin 910 in such a manner that space remains to accommodate the strut. The septal cartilage strut itself is fashioned so that it is slightly narrower than the medial crura and conforms to their curvature (Fig. 66). Its lower end should be rounded and its upper end tapered so that it extends no higher than the level of the upper border of the nostrils. It is fixed in place with sutures.

5. If the lateral crura need rotation, a triangular wedge of cartilage, base directed cephalically, is excised from each hinge area; on the other hand, if the lateral crura need to be shortened, rectangles of various sizes may be removed from the same areas (Fig. 67).

6. Final trimming of the medial ends of the lateral crura is not done until the mucous membrane beneath them and behind the upper ends of the medial crura have been stitched together over the caudal end of the septal dorsum. Suturing accomplishes three things: it eliminates a potential dead space in the supratip area, brings together the upper ends of the medial crura, and provides increased projection and support for the medial ends of the lateral crura. The lateral crura are now trimmed so that each crus abuts two structures, the ipsilateral medial crus and the contralateral crus in the midline (Fig. 68).

7. Cartilage implants are introduced, if necessary. Those over the lateral crura and in the supratip area are morselized to conform better to the underlying surface.

8. The retracted skin is replaced over the lobule and the columella, and the transcolumellar incision and rim incisions are closed with 6–0 polypropylene. The end of a blunt periosteal elevator is inserted to tent the skin overlying the lobular cartilages so that they might assume their proper positions.

9. If a shield graft is used, it is inserted as the last step of the operation through one of the columella rim incisions. It extends from the tip of the nose down to the transcolumella incision (Fig. 69).

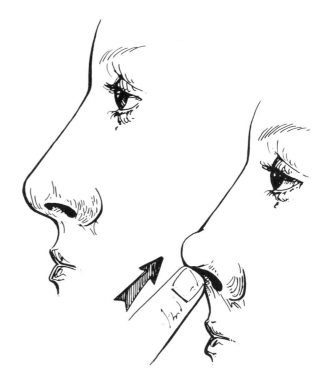

Figure 45. Pressing the columella against the caudal ends of the septum will reveal how much the nose can be shortened by modifying the lateral crura alone.

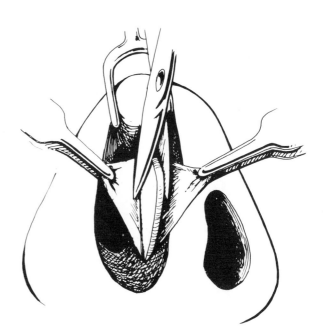

Figure 46. The caudal end of the septum should not be shortened arbitrarily; it should be reserved for the few cases which rotation of the tip cartilages produces insufficient shortening of the length of the dorsum.

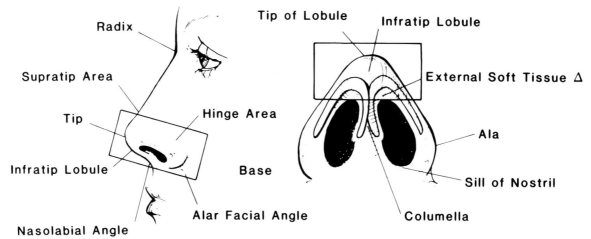

Figure 47.   Nasal base nomenclature.

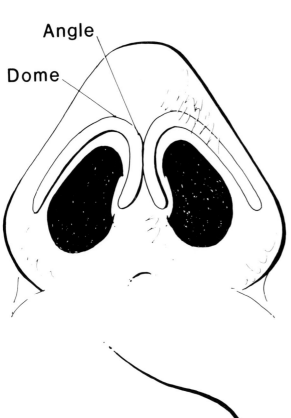

Figure 48.   The angle of an alar cartilage is where the medial and lateral crura meet. The dome is formed by the medial end of the lateral crus and is always lateral to the angle. Surgery usually attempts to move the dome closer to the angle.

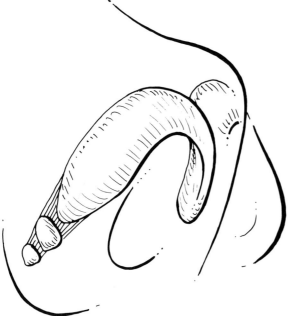

Figure 49.   The hinge of the lateral crus is the flexible part of the cartilage that sinks inward when the nasal base is rotated upward; it is located between the body of the cartilage and the accessory cartilages or its lateral continuation.

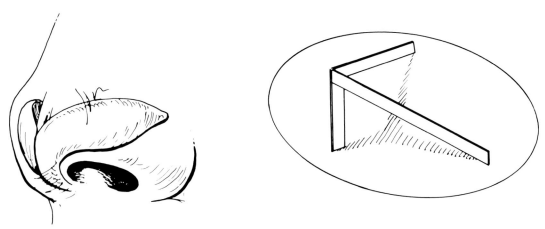

Figure 50. Similarity between the lower lateral cartilages and a tripod. The conjoined medial crura form one short leg of the tripod, and the lateral crura form the other two legs.

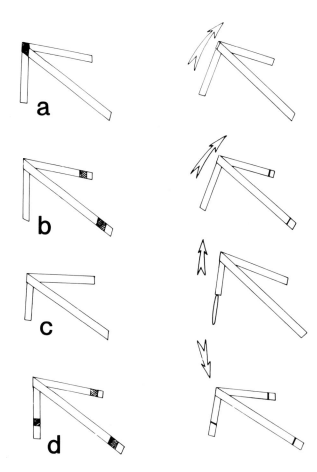

Figure 51. a: Shortening the medial ends of the lateral crura rotates the tip. b: Shortening the lateral ends of the lateral crura also permits tip rotation. c: Increasing the length of the medial crura increases tip projection and causes slight rotation. d: Decreasing the length of both the medial and lateral crura decreases tip projection.

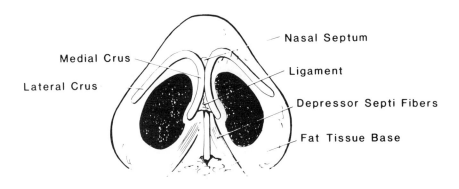

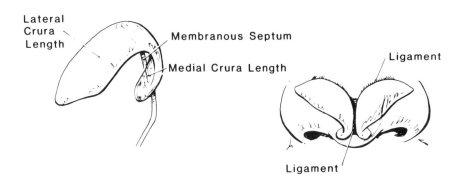

Figure 52. Supports of the nasal base of the tripod. The most important ones are the septal dorsum and the medial crura-caudal septum overlap.

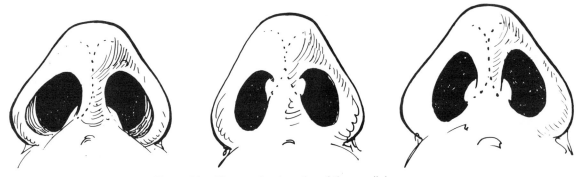

Figure 53.   The varying lengths of the medial crura.

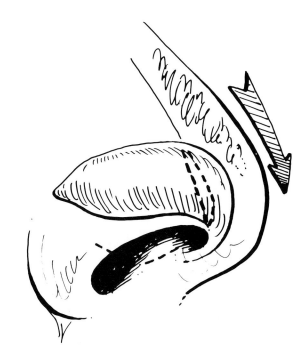

Figure 54. When the lateral crura are left too long at the end of the rhinoplasty, they push the tip downward during healing and cause hypertrophic scar tissue accumulation in the supratip area, a so-called soft tissue polly beak deformity.

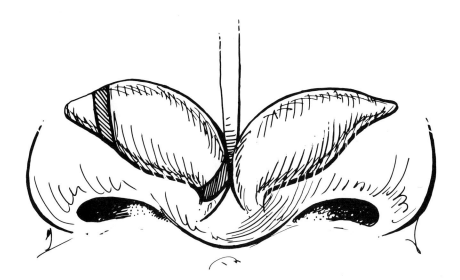

Figure 55. Methods of shortening the lateral crura: from the hinge areas and from the medial ends after the alar cartilages have been divided at their angles. Both methods permit tip rotation.

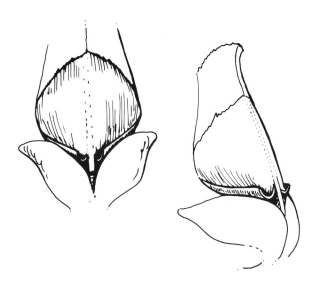

Figure 56. "Returning" of the upper lateral cartilages.

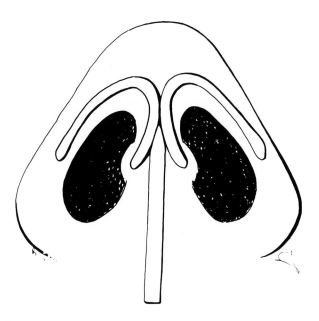

Figure 57. Shoring strut of septal cartilage used to maintain tip projection when the medial crura are of insufficient length to do so. It extends from about the level of the nostril apexes to within 2 mm of the premaxillary crest.

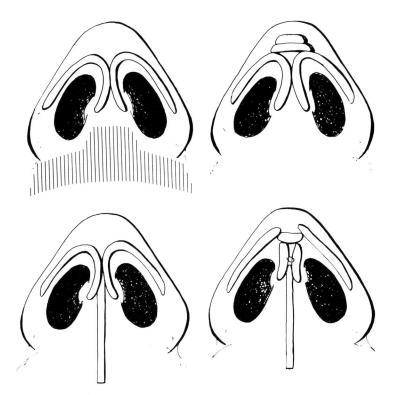

Figure 58. Methods of increasing tip projection. Upper left: Undermining premaxillary skin and soft tissue and moving it into the columella base. Upper right: Onlay grafts. Lower left: Intracrural strut. Lower right: Increasing length of medial crura.

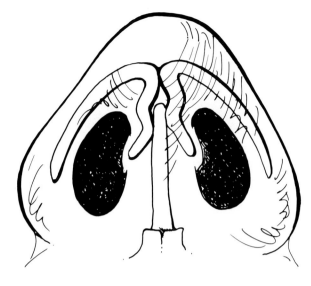

Figure 59.   Buckling of the upper ends of the medial crura due to developmental tensions caused by the lateral crura. The alar cartilages should be divided at their angles in such cases so that the lateral crura tension will not distort the lobule.

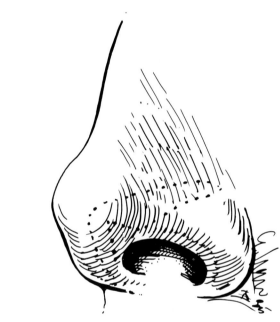

Figure 60.   Acute angulation that occurs in alar cartilages when cartilage tensions are not released. These angulations result in skin projections called "knuckling" or "knobbing." They are often seen when intact rim techniques are used inappropriately.

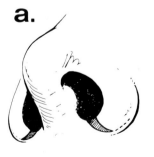

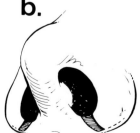

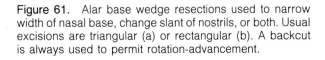

Figure 61.   Alar base wedge resections used to narrow width of nasal base, change slant of nostrils, or both. Usual excisions are triangular (a) or rectangular (b). A backcut is always used to permit rotation-advancement.

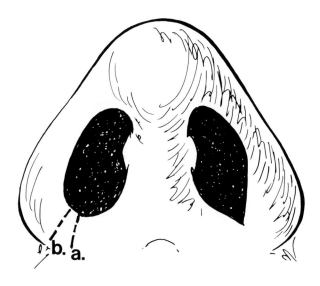

Figure 62. When wedge resections are made from the sill of the nostrils, the incisions should always preserve a bit of the curvature of the lower part of the lateral nostril wall; otherwise, the lower part of the nostril will be pointed instead of round.

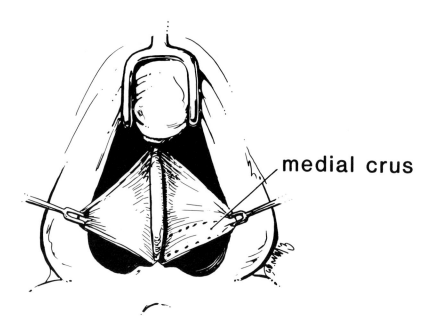

medial crus

Figure 63. Separation of the domes of the alar cartilages in external rhinoplasty.

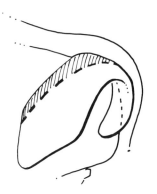 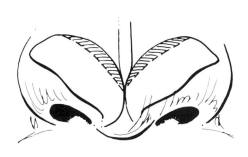

Figure 64. Excision of the scrolls. The excision should continue downward into the upper ends of the medial crura if they are widened.

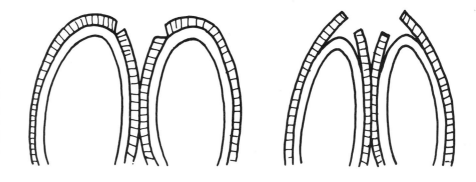

Figure 65. Dissecting the underlying vestibular skin from the medial ends of the lateral crura will cause them to straighten and increase their projection; the same is true of the medial crura to a lesser extent.

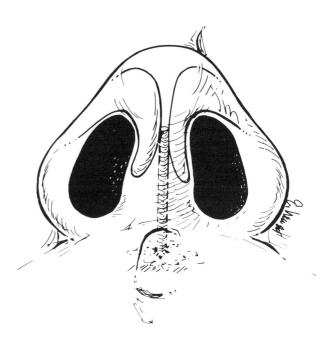

Figure 66. Placement of the cartilage strut between the medial crura to increase their length.

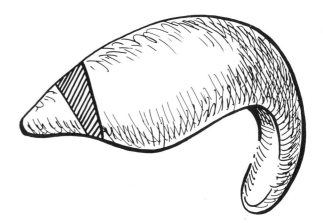

Figure 67. Configuration of cartilage excision from lateral reaches of lateral crus when tip rotation is desired; it resembles a truncated triangle, base directed cephalically.

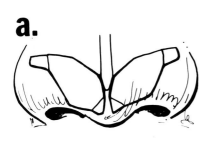

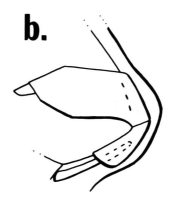

Figure 68. When the alar cartilages are cut at the angles and trimmed to remodel the lobule, the medial ends of the lateral crura should not only abut the medial crura, but should also abut each other in the midline.

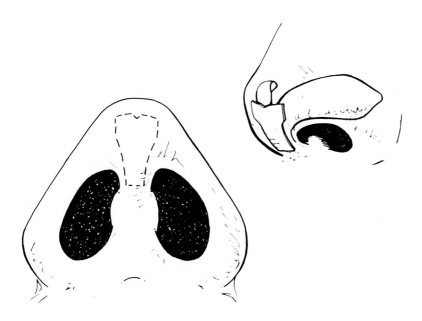

Figure 69. The shield graft. It is used to recontour the infratip lobule area, if necessary.

12   The Nasal Septum and Rhinoplasty

If the nose is thought of as resembling an A-frame building with a central wall (the septum) that meets the converging side walls, it should be obvious that the septum might become an important factor in any rhinoplasty. Actually, one of the following conditions may be encountered:

1.   A straight nose without septal disease
2.   A straight nose with septal disease that causes symptoms or would interfere with successful performance of rhinoplasty
3.   Deviation of only the cartilagenous part of the external nose; this always implies deviation of the underlying septum
4.   Crookedness of both the bony and cartilagenous vaults of the pyramid

For surgical purposes, it is convenient to divide the septum into two parts, an anterior portion underlying the nasal pyramid and a posterior segment (Fig. 70). Distortions of the deeper segment do not affect the appearance of the nose; they can be managed during rhinoplasty by traditional submucous resection without adversely affecting the shape of the external nose or jeopardizing its support. However, deflection of the anterior section usually causes external distortion; if not, it might interfere with narrowing the pyramid during operation.

When the two operations are indicated, that is, rhinoplasty and septal correction, the surgeon must know how to combine them; staging is unnecessary if one is a proficient nasal surgeon, but straightening some noses can become a *tour de force* for even the most skillful. Consequently, a bit of hedging often is in order; patients with marked deviation should be warned in advance that a secondary touch-up procedure of lesser magnitude may be required.

SURGICAL ANATOMY

The nasal septum consists of the following parts (Fig. 71):

1.   The quadrangular cartilage
2.   The medial crura of the alar cartilages
3.   The crests of the nasal bones
4.   The perpendicular plate of the ethmoid bone
5.   The vomer
6.   The maxillary crest
7.   The premaxillary alae
8.   The nasal spine
9.   The membranous septum

These structures are covered by a mucosal layer of mucoperichondrium and mucoperiosteum. The layer is continuous except where the caudal border of the quadrangular cartilage articulates with part of the vomer, the maxillary crest, the premaxillary alae, and the nasal spine.

Septal Cartilage

This cartilage is quadrangular in shape. From its ventral border (also called the cartilagenous dorsum), the upper lateral cartilages diverge like wings extending lateralward toward the piriform margins to form the upper cartilagenous vault of the external nose (Fig. 72); this conjoint arrangement extends upward for a few millimeters beneath the caudal end of the bony vault, and the lower ends of the upper lateral cartilages are overlapped by the alar cartilages that are sometimes referred to as the lower cartilagenous vault.

Part of the ventral edge of the septum is widened and even grooved at times. This is of interest from the standpoint of the width of the angle the upper lateral cartilages make with the septum; their caudal ends, which form the so-called nasal valve, create angles of 10°; the angles increase to 40° where the septal dorsum widens.

The caudal border of the septal cartilage presents a free margin that has superior and inferior angles. The caudal ends of the upper lateral cartilages always stop 4 mm or more proximal to the superior angle, and the nasal spine rarely extends to the inferior angle; both facts have surgical significance when nasal shortening is contemplated. The remainder of the caudal border is normally joined to the nasal spine, premaxillary alae, and maxillary crest in a tongue and groove arrangement; it sits in a mucoperichondrial sling that is, in turn, is fused with the periosteal covering of the bones.

The quadrangular cartilage joins the perpendicular plate of the ethmoid superiorly and the vomer posteroinferiorly. In addition, a narrow strip extends posteriorly on one side of the vomer, reaching to the face of the sphenoid bone at times; it is an important component of the septal spurring frequently found at the vomeroethmoid junction.

Septal cartilage is very flexible, yields easily to pressure during development or from trauma and is involved in almost every nasal deformity; incidentally, bent cartilage often straightens when deformities of the bones to which it is attached are corrected.

Medial Crura

Though the medial crura are not usually thought of as being part of the septal partition, undeniably they are. Joined together by fibrous tissue loosely termed a "ligament," their inferior ends overlap the caudal free border of the septum in a tongue and groove arrangement that constitutes an important support of the nasal tip. Their length varies, so tip projection can be decreased considerably in some cases by excising underlying septal cartilage to destroy the supportive overlap.

Nasal Crests

This small component of the septum is formed of inner extensions of the medial borders of the nasal bones; they articulate with the perpendicular plate of the ethmoid, the frontal spine, and, sometimes, with the quadrangular cartilage. If not in the midline, they can cause septal straightening and pyramid narrowing to become very difficult.

Perpendicular Plate of the Ethmoid Bone

The perpendicular plate meets the crests of the nasal bones, as already noted, and it has important articulations with the vomer and the septal cartilage. Since fusion of its ossifying centers does not occur until the 17th year, it is at the mercy of tensions created during enlargement of the face and transmitted upward through the other septal elements. Fortunately, it is a thin bone that can be easily cut into segments for safe piecemeal removal.

Vomer

Like the septal cartilage, the vomer is quadrangular in shape. Its ventral border meets the perpendicular plate of the ethmoid, and it is grooved anteriorly to receive the septal cartilage; the anterior end of the groove is continuous with the groove atop the maxillary crest that extends past the premaxillae to the nasal spine. The caudal border of the vomer abuts the posterior part of the crest of the maxilla and the palatine bones. Noteworthy is the fact that the mucoperiosteum may be elevated in one sheet over the perpendicular plate and vomer and that the mucoperichondrial sling surrounding the caudal border of the septal cartilage loses its integrity as the deeper reaches of the vomerine groove are approached.

Vomerine ossification begins early. As noted previously, the bone exerts vertical pressure on the perpendicular plate of the ethmoid and through the septal cartilage to the nasal dorsum development of the lower half of the face. Considerable spur formation is often found where the vomer and perpendicular plate meet.

Premaxillary Alae

The lips of the groove atop the maxillary crest usually widen as it approaches the nasal spine; sometimes, they must be removed to narrow the base of the septum and improve the patency of the internal nares. The wideness is caused by the alae of the premaxillae, bones that fuse with the maxillae during development. Continuous elevation of the nasal mucosa in this area without tearing is difficult.

Nasal Spine

The spine is a prominent projection of the maxillae in the midsagittal plane. It is roughly pyramidal in shape, varies in length, but rarely reaches the inferior septal angle and usually has a sharp edge along its lower surface. The upper surface is grooved for reception of the septal cartilage for which it provides important support.

Membranous Septum

The only part of the septum without a skeletal framework is the interval between the caudal end of the quadrangular cartilage and the medial crura; it consists of apposed nasal lining only. The area, appropriately called the membranous septum, widens as it proceeds upward toward the nasal tip from the point where the lower ends of the crura overlap the septal cartilage; the upper end forms the internal soft triangle that spans the hiatus between the medial and lateral crura. The membranous septum allows mobility of the base of the nose and the nasal tip; scarring in the area restricts movement and may contribute to gradual changes in the appearance of the postoperative nose.

TIMING OF SEPTAL SURGERY

We recommend that septal correction follow hump removal during septorhinoplasty for several reasons:

1. Surgical exposure of the septum is improved, especially when the open approach is used
2. Uncapping the dorsum will sometimes allow bent cartilage to straighten
3. To ensure that a wide septal support is left beneath the dorsum
4. To forestall the possiblity of accidentally disarticulating the subjacent perpendicular plate-cartilage junction.

SURGICAL TECHNIQUE

Exposure

Since mucosal junction tunnels have already been created to permit intramucosal hump removal (Chapter 13), one need only widen the elevation to gain access to sites requiring septal modification.

The extent of mucosal elevation depends on how much septal work is contemplated. If correction of only the posterior segment is planned, the mucosa is elevated from both sides of that area but left attached to one side of the anterior segment (Fig. 73). When both sectors require straightening, the membranes are elevated in their entirety from both sides of the skeleton. One need not fear that they will fall into the nose because they remain attached to the upper lateral cartilages and undersurface of the nasal bones (Fig. 73b).

Mucosal elevation is not difficult over the quadrangular cartilage, the perpendicular plate, and most of the vomer unless one encounters fracture adhesions, cartilage overlaps, or scarring; in such cases, the dissection is first carried above and below the bound-down areas. More difficulty is encountered where the mucoperichondrial sling of the cartilage fuses with the mucoperiosteal covering of the nasal spine, premaxillary alae, and

maxillary crest (Fig. 74). It can be facilitated if, after correcting the deformity of the posterior segment, the base of the remaining caudal buttress of cartilage is separated from the underlying bone (spine, premaxillary alae) and swung aside to expose the grooved area atop the bones where the fusion exists. Using the edges of the groove as a guide, the fused area is cut with a fine-pointed iris scissors to establish continuity of elevation with the periosteal covering of the bony base of the septum. As an alternative, the maxilla-premaxilla approach of Cottle can be used: a second compartment is made by elevating the mucoperiosteum along the floor of the nose and base of the septum; the areas of elevation are then made confluent.

It is almost impossible not to lacerate the membranes during their elevation, particularly over spurs, grooves, or when there is sharp angulation or an old fracture; it is particularly difficult when performing secondary septorhinoplasty. Unopposed lacerations of one side are usually of no lasting consequence because they heal rapidly, even if not sutured or if tissue has been lost. However, a permanent septal perforation may ensue when lacerations of both sides face each other; after carefully closing each opening with sutures, a plate of cartilage should be inserted between them.

Killian-Type Submucous Resection

The first incision through the septal cartilage is made with the 45° angle of a Rosen tympanoplasty flap knife; it parallels the caudal free border, begins about 1.5 cm from the dorsal border, and ends by transecting the thickened inferior margin of the quadrangular plate a few millimeters deep to the base of the nasal spine and piriform opening (Fig. 75). Bony support of the caudal septum is thereby preserved.

A second, slanting incision (Fig. 75b) beginning at the junction of the quadrangular cartilage with the perpendicular plate is made with a no. 15 blade to join the upper end of the first cut. Thus, a tapered strip of septal cartilage measuring about 8 mm wide above at the perpendicular plate-cartilage junction and 12 to 15 mm below remains beneath the nasal dorsum and forms a continuous L-shaped buttress with the cartilage remaining behind the columella.

Tapering the cephalic end of the dorsal buttress ensures sufficient space, if it does not exist, for later infracture of the bony lamina. If there is enough space, the dorsal buttress is made the same width along its entire course.

Next, the superior border of the cartilage segment to be removed is separated from the perpendicular plate with the tympanoplasty knife (Fig. 75c) all the way to the vomeroethmoid junction. The inferior edge of the cartilage can now be easily elevated from the maxillary crest-vomerine groove and removed (Fig. 75d).

We do not hesitate to remove relatively large pieces of septal cartilage because there will be no loss of external pyramid support provided wide dorsal and caudal buttresses have been left in situ (Fig. 76). Neither have we found it necessary to replace pieces of cartilage between the mucosal flaps to forestall postoperative flaccidity because that has not been a problem; meticulous elevation of perichondrium and periosteum may play a part in preventing this complication.

Deflected portions of the perpendicular plate are now removed up to the subradix area. To avert possible fracture of the cribiform plate, the bone is first cut into narrow strips with a Mayo scissors so that they can be extracted piecemeal (Fig. 77).

If deflection of the perpendicular plate extends anteriorly into the immediate subradix area, the dorsal buttress of septal cartilage is sewn to the cephalic ends of the upper lateral cartilages to prevent inward displacement later (Fig. 78). The perpendicular plate-quadrangular cartilage is divided, and then the offending deflection of the perpendicular plate can be removed. Portions of the nasal crest may have to be excised if they contribute to the deflection. Neither maneuver will result in collapse of the nasal bones.

Deformities of the vomer are treated in a similar manner.

Lipping of the maxillary crest can be removed with a Lempert rongeur, but, if the whole structure is deviated, it is cut along its base with an osteotome and removed, or it can be sculpted with a dental drill.

When the septal deformity is confined to the perpendicular plate, the vomer, the maxillary crest, or all three, the mucosa can be left attached to one side of the septum and the respective bones exposed and corrected through liberating incisions made around the periphery of the cartilage. This procedure is more difficult than what has already been described, but it does preserve the integrity of the quadrangular cartilage (Fig. 79).

The nasal cavities are not packed after a Killian submucous resection. This is possible because the mucosa is meticulously elevated and no blood vessels course between the septal flaps. If the inner surface of the mucosa is inadvertently nicked during surgery, the bleeding point is cauterized with a bipolar cautery; if further bleeding is feared, an incision can be made for drainage through one flap near the floor of the nose.

After submucous resection, several mattress sutures of 0000 plain catgut swedged to a short Keith needle (Ethicon no. 1828G) are used to coapt the mucosal flaps. Also, the completely mobilized septal flap is elevated and sutured to the remaining septal cartilage near the superior septal angle (Fig. 80).

We perform septal surgery of some type in about 95% of the rhinoplasties. Most are to provide functional improvement or to make pyramid straightening possible. However, some minimal procedures are done to provide sufficient space beneath the pyramid to achieve satisfactory narrowing.

Anterior Segment Septal Surgery

Deformities of the anterior segment take a variety of forms: bowing of the cartilage, eccentric placement of the perpendicular plate, or cartilage in the subradix area, angulation of varying degrees, thickening, deviation of the radix, or a combination of these. They are usually, but not always, associated with a deformity of the external nose. For example, a bowed septal cartilage may interfere with breathing but not produce an external deformity, or the cartilage may be dislocated from its bony base anteriorly but cause little more than columellar deviation.

When septal and external nasal deformities coexist, successful repair depends on recognition of their interdependence; neither can be adequately corrected alone.

Whatever the case, the mucosa is elevated from both sides of the anterior segment but left attached to the nasal bones and to upper lateral cartilages after they have been cut from the cartilagenous dorsum; the hump is removed and a Killian-type submucous resection of the posterior segment is performed, if needed, before attention is directed to the subpyramidal area.

Bowing of the cartilage can often be treated effectively by morselization, provided it is done properly. This implies that the jaws of the instrument are applied to both sides of the cartilage over the entire area of the bend, that they are closed gradually and tightly, that the force is maintained for several seconds instead of briefly, and that the pliant cartilage produced is splinted in the midline for at least a week; it takes at least that long for its rigidity to be reconstituted. Using morselization on only one side of a piece of cartilage has proved to be unreliable in our hands, possibly because the attached mucoperichondrium is a limiting factor. Finally, it should be remembered that cartilage expands as a result of morselization, so trimming is usually required to make it fit properly.

We have little confidence in crosshatching one side of a plate of bowed septal cartilage to cause it to straighten, whether or not its mucoperichondrium is attached. However, curved narrow strips can be straightened fairly well by making several superficial transverse incisions across their concave surfaces.

Correction of *eccentric location of the nasal crest* has been discussed previously.

Deviation of the radix means that three structures are off-center: the solid upper ends of the two nasal bones and the frontal spine. Fortunately, this deformity is relatively rare because we know of no technique whereby they can be separated and precisely modified so that they will assume a midline position. When encountering it, we have attempted to handle the condition by carefully and progressively sculpting the complex with small osteotomes and narrow rongeurs or a motor-driven burr. Before doing this, however, the underlying septum must be separated from the radix.

Even if the entire radix is removed, the nasal bones will not fall backward into the nasal cavity. Their rigidity and hip joint configuration prevents this. Some deepening of the nasofrontal angle may occur; however, it can be corrected with one or more cartilage implants.

Correction of radix deviation can be facilitated considerably by using the open rhinoplasty approach; even then, it remains difficult nasal surgery.

Angulation of the anterior segment may be confined to septal cartilage, may occur where the cartilage meets the perpendicular plate, may be due to deviaton of the radix, or may be caused by any combination of these things.

The only reliable way to correct angulations of the cartilage or those found where the cartilage joins the perpendicular plate is to remove a complete strip of cartilage at the bend. The danger is that the distal buttress will become free-floating unless the caudal cartilage remains firmly attached to the nasal spine and premaxillary alae, a happy state seldom found because that union must also be disrupted as a rule.

Several steps are taken to prevent displacement of the distal cartilage:

1. Transseptal mattress sutures are inserted beneath the dorsal buttress of cartilage to prevent it from falling into the nose after division has been completed. The upper end of each suture passes through cartilage and the lower one through membrane·only (Fig. 81). Ethicon septal suture (no. 1828G) is ideal for this purpose

2. Likewise, one or more mattress sutures are passed through the cartilage distal to the angulation

3. The cartilagenous dorsum caudal to the bend is sutured to the upper lateral cartilages

4. If a preliminary "swinging-door" procedure has been performed, the inferior border of the caudal buttress is fixed in the midline with two Wright sutures, similar to those previously described to support the dorsal buttress

5. A cartilage strut is placed between the medial crura and extended downward below the nasal spine almost to the premaxilla to guard against possible columella retraction (Fig. 82).

6. Septocolumellar sutures are inserted

7. The previously mobilized caudal end of the septum is splinted with exposed x-ray film

8. The lateral walls of the pyramid have been mobilized so that they can act as splints after the nose has been narrowed and the external dressing applied

It is evident that interruption of the dorsal continuity should be the last step of rhinoplasty.

Nasal spine deformities, fortunately, can be corrected by partial excision so that its septal supportive function is not compromised (Fig. 83). The true extent of spinal deformity often cannot be judged until the structure is skeletonized by cutting away the periosteum and muscles attached to it.

Upper lateral cartilage asymmetry frequently accompanies long-standing deformities of the anterior septal segment. After the pyramid has been centered, one cartilage may be longer than the other and project above the septal dorsum; the excess must be excised to equalize the structures. Even when asymmetry is not so obvious, we find it helpful to undermine a few millimeters of mucosa from beneath the medial borders of the cartilage.

The nasal bones may, also, be asymmetric, causing one of them to project above the dorsal profile after the pyramid has been straightened. That excess must, also, be excised. A double lateral osteotomy will lessen the amount of bone in excess and, often, will obviate the need for excising any bone.

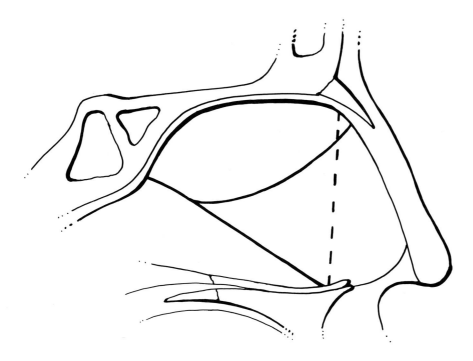

Figure 70. Division of the nasal septum into anterior and posterior portions for surgical purposes. The posterior portion can usually be modified with impunity during rhinoplasty.

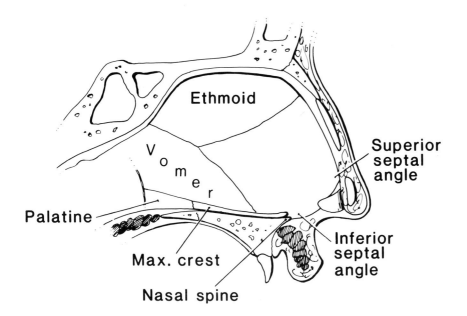

Ethmoid

Superior septal angle

Vomer

Palatine

Inferior septal angle

Max. crest

Nasal spine

Figure 71. The components of the nasal septum. Most of them may have to be modified when correcting a twisted nose.

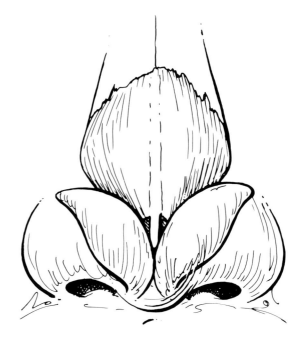

Figure 72. The upper lateral cartilages are winglike lateral extensions of the nasal dorsum; they extend for a few millimeters beneath the caudal ends of the nasal bones superiorly and beneath the scrolls of the lower lateral cartilages inferiorly.

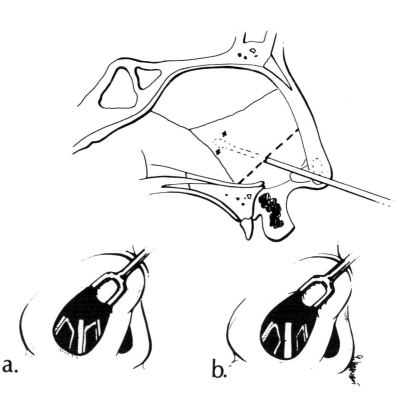

Figure 73. a: When only the posterior segment of the septum is to be straightened, the mucosa may be left attached to one side of the anterior segment. b: The mucosa is elevated bilaterally when the entire septum must be straightened. Its attachment to the upper lateral cartilages prevents it from falling into the interior of the nose.

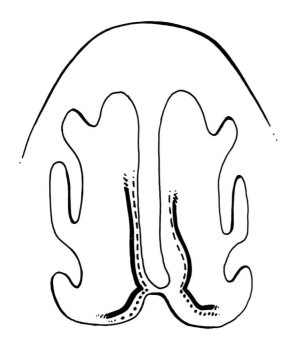

Figure 74. Making the mucoperichondrial sling of the septal cartilage continuous with the mucoperiosteal covering of the nasal spine, premaxillary alae, and the anterior part of the maxillary crest. Mucosal tears often occur if this is not done carefully.

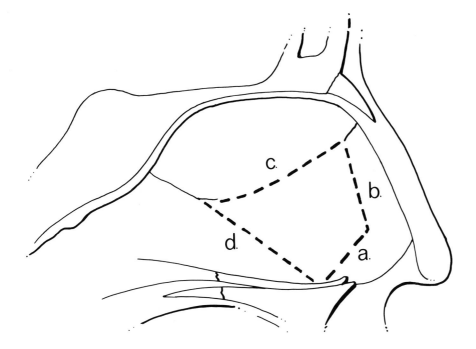

Figure 75. Incisions made through the septal cartilage for a Killian-type submucous resection. See text for details.

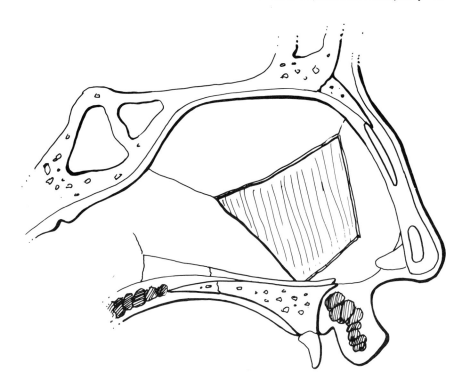

Figure 76. Wide dorsal and caudal buttresses of cartilages left intact after Killian-type submucous resection. This causes no loss of external pyramid support.

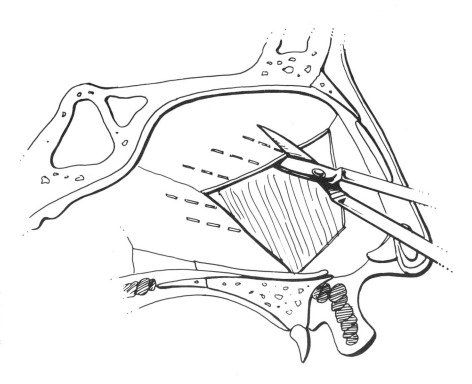

Figure 77. A method of removing the bones of the septum in a piecemeal fashion; in the case of a deviated ethmoid, this lessens the possibility of fracturing the cribiform plate.

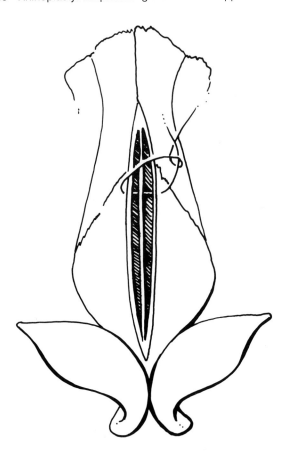

Figure 78. Anchoring the septal cartilage to the upper lateral cartilages to forestall inward displacement when the continuity of the dorsal cartilage buttress with the perpendicular plate of the ethmoid must be interrupted to straighten the nose. This is very easy to do when the external approach is used.

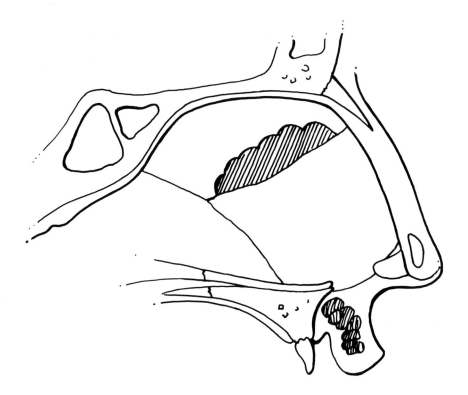

Figure 79. It is possible to remove parts of the ethmoid and/or vomer without removing any of the quadrangular cartilage.

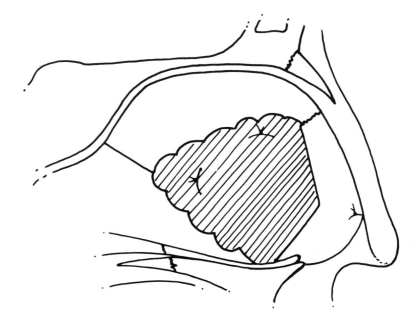

Figure 80. After submucous resection, the mucosal flaps are coapted with mattress sutures. If the membranes have been elevated *in toto* from both sides, the membranes are sutured to the septal cartilage at the superior septal angle.

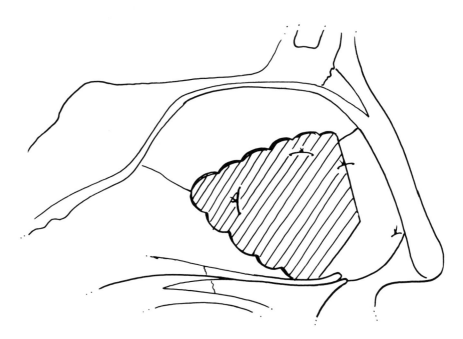

Figure 81. When the continuity of the dorsal bony-cartilagenous buttress must be interrupted to straighten a deviated pyramid, transseptal mattress sutures may be used to prevent displacement of the cartilage inward.

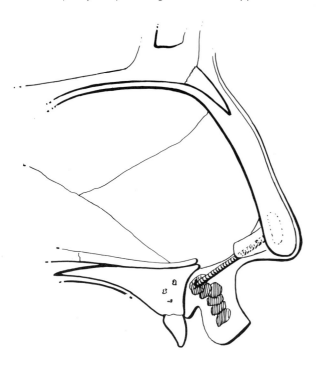

Figure 82. A cartilage strut placed between the medial crura and extended downward below the nasal spine helps prevent entad displacement of loosened septal cartilage and columellar retraction.

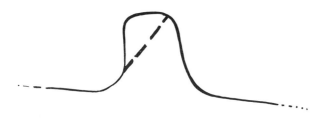

Figure 83. Rather than fracturing the nasal spine at its base to achieve straightening, we find that trimming it with a McIndoe bone-cutting forceps is effective; cutting the spine on a bias instead of fracturing it maintains its supportive function.

13   Hump Removal

The amount of hump to be removed or dorsal augmentation necessary should be estimated during preoperative planning (Chapter 6). The two landmarks that are important in planning hump removal are the nasofrontal angle and the projection of the nasal tip. Any part of the skeleton projecting above a line connecting them should be leveled (Fig. 84); conversely, to correct a saddle nose, the dorsum has to be built up to meet the line.

Sometimes, the landmarks themselves have to be altered to achieve the desired profile. For example, the nasofrontal angle may have to be deepened or augmented; likewise, the tip may need to be rotated and its projection increased or decreased. An inverse relationship exists between tip projection and the amount of hump removal needed, and vice versa. Nasofrontal angle modification will affect hump removal in a similar manner; if it is deepened, more hump will have to be removed; if augmented, less hump will need to be removed.

When a shallow nasofrontal angle is due to thickening of the procerus muscle, the muscle can be avulsed with a narrow Lempert rongeur or similar stout forceps; it is important not to overlook the lateral parts of the muscles, or the root of the nose might appear too wide postoperatively. If shallowness is due to a superabundance of bone, the excess can be removed with the technique described later in this chapter.

A deep nasofrontal angle may occur alone or as part of a saddle nose deformity. In either event, we use septal cartilage implants obtained from the patient's septum or from the cartilage bank to correct the condition; the cartilage is morselized or crushed so that it conforms to the contour of the underlying bone.

Finally, one should distinguish between a naturally occurring hump and one that appears after supratip saddling caused by trauma or infection, among others. Very little hump removal may be indicated in such cases if the profile was relatively satisfactory before the incident; insertion of cartilage implants into the depression often corrects the condition satisfactorily.

PERTINENT SURGICAL ANATOMY

The skeletal composition of the nasal dorsum is well known. Not generally appreciated, however, is the fact that, even when the profile is aesthetically pleasing, the underlying skeleton describes a gentle convexity whose high point is located at the rhinion (Fig. 85). The overlying skin is thinnest at that point, and the soft tissue covering gradually thickens above and below the rhinion to make the profile attractive. Wright pointed out that the thickness of the soft-tissue covering should be considered during hump removal and that the surgical aim should be to reproduce nature. He showed that straight-line hump removal results in a low point in the profile where the skin is thinnest, making it appear as though the nasofrontal angle has been moved caudally (Fig. 86). To avert this, the cartilagenous dorsum should be secondarily lowered, beginning at the rhinion, to accommodate the gradual thickening of the overlying tissues. This, also, helps to minimize the development of another untoward sequela, the cartilagenous polly beak deformity.

INSTRUMENTATION AND APPROACH

We have used a variety of instruments for hump removal: scissors and scalpels for the cartilagenous portions; saws, flat osteotomes, bone-cutting forceps and scissors, rasps, and motor-driven burrs for the bony section. Whatever instrument is used, we always perform hump removal intramucosally, that is, without cutting the mucosa beneath any part of the hump; this is done by creating mucosal tunnels beneath the hump before its removal is started (Fig. 87). Our aim is to decrease bleeding and to avoid the possibility of adverse scar tissue contracture and other sequelae. Mucosal redundancy has never posed a problem postoperatively; it seems to shrink to conform to its new surroundings.

We prefer retrograde hump removal, that is, to work upward from the caudal end. However, neither the approach nor the instruments used are as important as preciseness and a smooth dorsum afterward.

OPERATIVE STEPS

1. Mucosal tunnels are created beneath the junction of the nasal septum with the upper lateral cartilages and nasal bones.
2. The septal dorsum is lowered in small increments from the rhinion to its caudal end; in effect, a triangular piece of cartilage whose base is located caudally is excised. This makes the area of the rhinion more prominent (Fig. 88).
3. The bony hump may now be removed according to the preference of the surgeon:
   a. With a saw in the traditional manner: a straight Joseph saw remains best for this purpose.
   b. With a rasp (Fig. 89): We prefer an instrument with two tungsten carbide cutting surfaces, one that cuts on the upstroke and one that cuts on the downstroke; we find we can be more precise when removing bone with a push rasp. Incidentally, purchase with any rasp can be improved by creating shallow kerfs along the bony dorsum with a straight Joseph saw.
4. With a bone-biting forceps (Kazanjian, Goldman, or McIndoe). These are better used after the lateral walls have been separated from the septum.
5. With a flattened Rish or Rubin osteotome (Fig. 90), one must be careful not to allow these instruments to go off track.
6. With a motor-driven burr (Fig. 91), this becomes an easy and safe procedure, with the exposure provided by external rhinoplasty.

When the bony pyramid is deviated from the midline, the amount of hump to be removed is gauged on the narrow nasal wall, the convex side. Then any excess bone and upper lateral cartilage is excised from the wide side after the pyramid has been centered.

Secondary lowering of the cartilagenous dorsum is not done until after the pyramid has been narrowed and it has been determined that the supratip soft tissues will drape properly. One way of estimating how much additional lowering is necessary is to palpate the surpatip dorsum while the nostrils are being depressed toward the premaxilla (Fig. 92). As a general rule, the cartilage should be shaved until it lies about 2 mm above the level of the apexes of the nostrils; this assures sufficient tip projection to create the desired slight supratip depression, provided, of course, that columellar support is firm enough to resist postoperative settling.

After hump removal, one is well-advised to "sweep" the area and the undersurface of the overlying skin with a Maltz pull rasp to remove any bony or cartilagenous debris that may have been left behind, because these can become troublesome later. It is also well to pass the tip of a gloved finger that has been wet along the dorsum to search for irregularities of the bone or upper lateral cartilages.

If the patient has very thin skin that makes even the normal amount of irregularity visible and palpable, the condition can be concealed by laying a strip of Gelfoam, Vicryl mesh, Supramid mesh or crushed cartilage along the entire dorsum.

DEEPENING THE NASOFRONTAL ANGLE

The easiest way to deepen the angle is to make it part of hump removal. The process is divided into three parts. First, bilateral cuts are made through the nasal bones at the desired level with a Neivert osteotome and extended upward along each side of the radix to score the bone (Fig. 91a). Then, a flat Rubin or Rish osteotome is introduced through the cuts and advanced upward to sever the septum from the undersurface of the hump and to enter the body of the radix; progress of the chisel is slowed and, finally, stopped by the thick bone. When this happens, the entire block of bone is lifted with the osteotome until it separates from the frontal bone at the nasofrontal suture line; it is then removed with a strong forceps.

As an alternative, the nasofrontal angle can be deepened with a motor-driven burr after preliminary removal of as much hump as possible to provide access to the area.

We have been singularly unimpressed with the use of so-called curved nasofrontal rasps.

Excessive thickness of the soft tissues in the supratip area can prevent satisfactory drapeage of the skin over the newly modified nasal skeleton and lead to an unaesthetic rounding of the area after operation, a soft tissue polly beak.

It is possible to improve the plasticity of this

type of skin by excising any excessive tissue from the undersurface of the dermis, a structure easily distinguished by its color and consistency. When the need for removal is recognized before operation, the way to handle the situation is to keep the plane of dissection as close to the dermis as possible when elevating the tissues from the cartilagenous structures (Fig. 93); subsequently, they can be dissected en bloc from the cartilage under direct vision and without difficulty during the remainder of the external rhinoplasty.

The other method consists of dissecting the tissues from the undersurface of the dermis after the modification of the skeleton has been completed, the skin having been elevated in the usual way, that is, by keeping the plane of dissection as close to the cartilage as possible. A small angulated scissors (Converse) is ideal for this purpose. After the area has been exposed, an assistant puts traction on the excess tissue with a Brown-Adson thumb forceps to facilitate dissection with the scissors whose blades are always directed parallel to the dermis.

Should excessive bleeding occur from vessels located on the undersurface of the dermis, it can be controlled by inserting a cotton tampon soaked with epinephrine for a few minutes or by judicious use of a wet-field bipolar cautery; too vigorous cauterization may cause skin necrosis.

If dissecting away the excess soft tissue does not produce satisfactory skin drapeage, one additional thing can be done. The undersurface of the exposed dermis can be crosshatched with a new no. 15 scalpel blade (Fig. 94). The crosshatching should extend over the entire lobular and supratip areas and must be performed gingerly on the undersurface of the finger-backed skin; to avoid cutting through the skin, the incisions should be stopped as soon as the margins gape. If properly performed, this technique usually produces dramatic results. We have never encountered any untoward problems with or after its use.

PERSONAL OBSERVATION

When the senior author first began to perform rhinoplasty during the early 1950s, excessive hump removal was rampant and thousands of patients walked the streets of our major cities with the stigmata it produced, such as the scooped-out nose, the ski-jump, the small turned up nose with the wide, flat look in the intercanthal area, various types of polly beak deformities. These gave this wonderful operation "bad press" and patients rebelled; even today, potential patients will say they do not want a short, turned-up nose, etc.

The excesses stemmed from the fact that the operation was not understood and was frequently done by rote: after the dorsal skeleton was uncovered, the septum was routinely shortened and, then, a considerable amount of bony hump was removed, no thought being given to the relationship of the nasal dorsum to the location and projection of the nasal tip.

Surgeons who lived through that era and gained sophistication will attest to the fact that they now remove far less hump and perform less septal shortening than they did formerly.

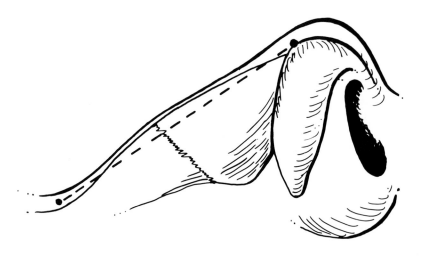

Figure 84. Landmarks important in determining how much nasal hump to remove. One or both may have to be changed before making a final decision.

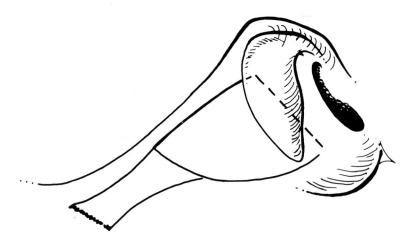

Figure 85. Skeletal profile of an aesthetically pleasing nose that should be replicated at the conclusion of rhinoplasty. NOTE: (1.) Rhinion is the high point of the skeletal profile; the overlying soft tissues are thinnest at this point; (2.) the soft tissues progressively thicken as the nasofrontal and superior septal angles are approached; and (3.) the tip of the nose projects several millimeters above the level of the superior septal angle.

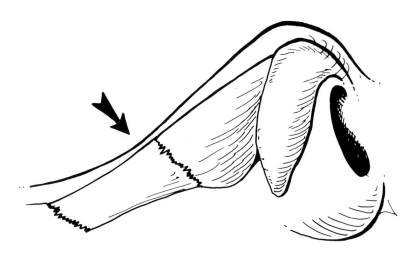

Figure 86. If the skeletal profile of the nose is left straight at the end of rhinoplasty, a concavity will result in the middorsal region, that is, the nose will appear scooped-out.

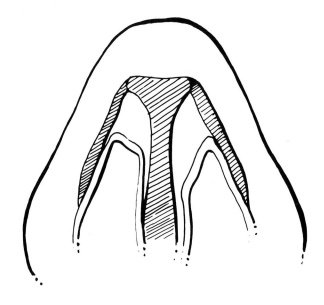

Figure 87. Mucosal tunnels created beneath the hump permit hump removal, medial osteotomies, and any septal surgery to be performed intramucosally, that is, without cutting the membranes; this procedure lessens operative bleeding and postoperative scar contractures.

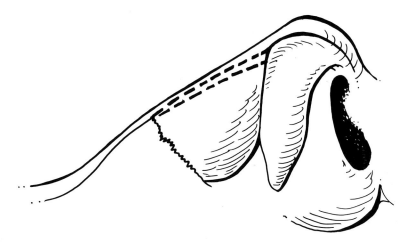

Figure 88. Incremental lowering of the cartilagenous dorsum makes the rhinion more prominent and facilitates hump removal.

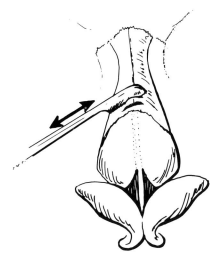

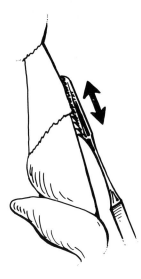

Figure 89. Hump removal with a rasp can be made easier by prior roughening of the bony dorsum with a straight Joseph saw and by using an instrument that cuts both on the upstroke and the downstroke (see text).

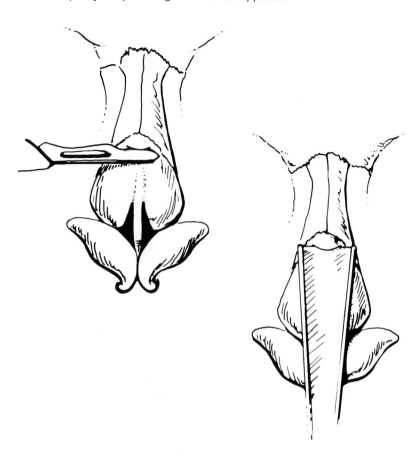

Figure 90. Although flattened osteotomes permit rapid hump removal, they must be carefully guided lest they stray from the intended course. Nicking the cartilagenous dorsum with a scalpel helps establish the proper depth at the start of the procedure.

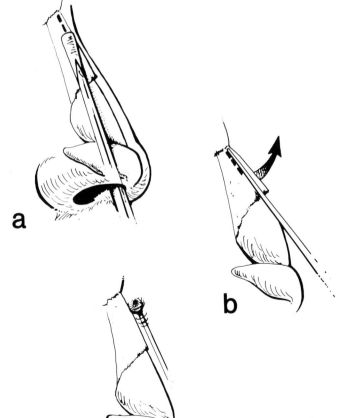

a

b

c

Figure 91. a, b: Deepening of the nasofrontal angle is made easier by scoring each side of the bony pyramid at the desired level with a Neivert osteotome before introducing a Rubin or Rish instrument. c: The contour of the bony dorsum can be accurately sculpted with a motor-driven burr when external rhinoplasty is performed.

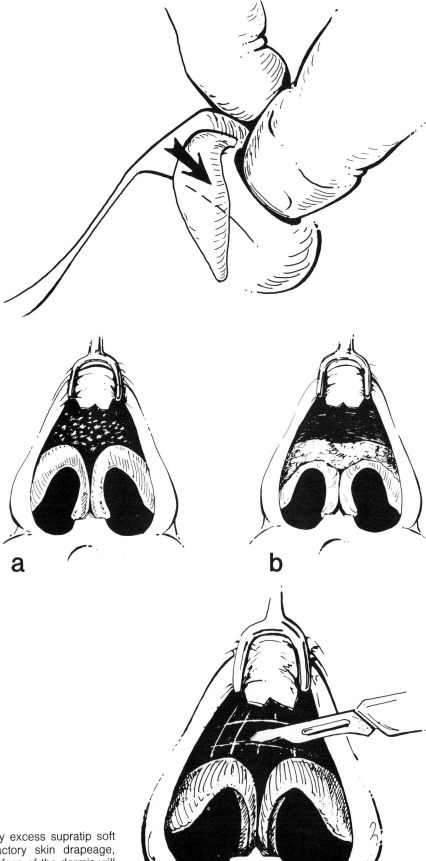

Figure 92. A method of determining how much secondary lowering of the cartilagenous dorsum is necessary before concluding rhinoplasty. The supratip dorsum is palpated while the nostrils are being depressed toward the premaxilla.

Figure 93. a: If thickened subcutaneous tissue overlying the tip cartilages and supratip area interfere with proper skin drapeage, it must be removed. b: Removal of the thickened soft tissue is facilitated by keeping the level of undermining close to the dermis when elevating the skin. The thick tissue remains attached to the alar cartilages and septal dorsum and can be removed in a safer and more thorough manner.

Figure 94. When dissecting away excess supratip soft tissue does not result in satisfactory skin drapeage, crosshatched cuts on the undersurface of the dermis will usually be effective. A fresh scalpel blade should be used and the skin should be finger-backed to prevent cutting too deeply.

14   Narrowing the Nose

The external nose is triangular in outline. Hump removal truncates the triangle below the level of the radix, converting it to a flat plane that must be subsequently narrowed for cosmetic purposes (Fig. 95).

Narrowing is accomplished by mobilizing the lateral walls and then moving them toward the septum. The walls are separated from each other and the septum by medial osteotomies, from the facial plane by lateral osteotomies, and from the radix by controlled fractures that join the cephalic ends of the medial and lateral osteotomies on each side.

Artistically, the aim is to cause the reconstructed dorsum to be about one-half as wide as the intercanthal distance and the new nasofacial angles to be tangential to lines dropped perpendicularly from the medial canthi (Fig. 96). Because these goals are frequently not reached, the rhinoplasty literature is replete with photographs wherein the noses look wider postoperatively than they did before operation.

PERTINENT ANATOMY

Hump removal partially separates the nasal bones from each other by creating a dehiscence in the nasal dorsum (Fig. 97). The length of the separation depends on how much hump is removed; the dehiscence is longer when large humps are removed, when they originate at the nasofrontal angle rather than farther inferiorly, and when the angle has been deepened. The higher it extends, the shorter will be the length of medial osteotomy needed; sometimes, none at all will be necessary.

The nasofacial grooves define the width of the nose and mark the junction of the frontal processes with the bodies of the maxillae. Each begins lateral to and at a deeper level than the piriform opening, and, together, they trace a pear-shaped configuration as they proceed upward. The frontal processes contribute less and less to the structure of the lateral nasal walls until their contribution becomes virtually nonexistent when the prelacrimal part of the grooves are reached.

An intimate knowledge of the structure of the radix nasi (also called the subglabellar segment and root of the nose) is helpful if one wants to avoid some of the pitfalls of nasal narrowing.

It is the thickest and strongest part of the external nose and consists of, from above downward, the nasal process of the frontal bone and the frontal spine, to which are firmly attached the dense upper ends of the nasal bones medially and the upper ends of the frontal processes of the maxillae laterally (Fig. 98).

Fortunately, the radix rarely needs narrowing; wideness of the nose is usually confined to the thin lateral walls caudal to it. Fortunately, too, the transformation from thick to thin bone is fairly abrupt, making it an ideal place to produce a controlled fracture uniting the upper ends of the medial and lateral osteotomies.

A thickened or deviated septum beneath the nasal pyramid can impede narrowing, so it is important to check in advance if there is enough room in the vault of the nose to permit infracturing the bones and moving them medialward; if not, the obstruction should be corrected.

OPERATIVE STEPS

1. Any attachment of the upper lateral cartilages to the septum that was not interrupted during hump removal is divided through the junction tunnels created for hump removal.
2. Short medial osteotomies are performed with a Mayo or Becker scissors; they follow the roof of the bony external nose and do not enter the radix.
3. An incision about 1 cm long is made along each piriform margin at the level of the anterior ends of each inferior turbinate.
4. The soft tissues adjacent to the piriform margin are bluntly elevated for a distance of about 5 mm with a sharp-pointed iris scissors.
5. Mucoperiosteal tunnels are created on

98

the inner and outer sides of each frontal process along the line of the proposed osteotomies.

6. Single or double osteotomies are performed with a straight Parkes osteotome.

7. Performance of the lateral osteotomies usually cause cephalic fractures to occur along the caudal ends of the lateral radix; if not, an attempt is made to produce them by medially directed thumb pressure against the lateral walls; if that is not successful, a Quisling shatter fracture osteotome is used.

8. After cephalic fractures have been created, the bones at the medial ends of each lateral wall are rasped to impact them closer to the underlying septum.

9. The septal dorsum and medial borders of the upper lateral cartilages are modified if they adversely affect narrowing.

MEDIAL OSTEOTOMY DETAILS

When medial osteotomy is necessary, it should always be done before lateral osteotomy.

The bones may be separated for the short distance necessary (Fig. 99) by successive snips made with the tips of a heavy Mayo or Becker scissors or by cuts made with a thin, flattened osteotome similar to the Rish or Rubin instruments that are commonly used for hump removal. In any event, the pathways should follow the roof of each nasal vault and not enter the body of the thick radix.

In that rare case when the radix itself needs narrowing, it should be sculpted from the outside; it is folly to believe that the solid structure can be narrowed by chisel kerfs, because they compress bone instead of excavating it. Attempting to narrow the radix by removing bone from its central core has not been successful in our hands and usually causes many vexations.

Entering the radix with an osteotome can produce a complication aptly called a "rocker" by Wright. The chisel may cause an angulated fracture that extends through the lateral wall of the solid upper part of the nasal bone (Fig. 100). When medially directed pressure is applied to narrow the widened dorsum, the entire lateral wall of the nose moves instead of only the lower thin portion. This causes the edge of the fracture to project from the side of the radix; when the fracture heals later, the lower part of the pyramid rewidens. In effect, the lateral nasal wall "rocks" on a fulcrum located at the lower end of the radix where the medial osteotomy should have stopped.

LATERAL OSTEOTOMY DETAILS

Moving the nasofacial angles medialward so that the base of the pyramid lies within the intercanthal boundaries is an integral part of most rhinoplasties. When their location is acceptable preoperatively, lateral osteotomies simply follow the underlying nasofacial grooves. When the base of the pyramid extends beyond the intercanthal boundaries, two osteotomies are performed on each side; the first is at a higher level on the frontal process and the second is lower down, in the nasofacial groove proper. These are popularly known as "double osteotomies" (Fig. 101).

The incisions made to introduce the Parkes osteotome are made at the level of the anterior ends of the inferior turbinates, because if nasal narrowing is started below this level, the airways may be compromised (Fig. 102). The cuts parallel the bony margin, are made only long enough to accommodate the instrument, and are made through vestibular skin because it seems to cause less bleeding than when made through mucosa.

The external periosteal tunnels extend along the nasofacial grooves until the upper reaches of the prelacrimal grooves are reached; they are made somewhat wider when double osteotomies are used. The internal tunnels are about two-thirds as long as the outer ones. This technique has two virtues. First, elevation of the membranes internally helps to avoid lacerating them with the chisel. Secondly, it provides leeway for movement of the bones where most is needed during nasal narrowing; however, it still maintains membrane attachment higher up to support the bones and foil possible displacement deep into the nose later during infracture.

When double osteotomies are used, the superficial ones are begun at the piriform margin and are directed straight upward toward the prelacrimal grooves; they delineate the new locations of the nasofacial grooves. The lower osteotomies are made in the nasofacial grooves; the chisel must first be directed toward the face from the piriform margin to reach the grooves before it can be turned cephalward (Fig. 103).

There are other items of interest about lateral osteotomies. The first relates to their length. They always extend to a higher level than the medial ones. This means that the fracture line that connects their upper ends should be directed obliquely, the lower border of the radix being the fulcrum along which the fracture occurs. This is contrary to the illustrations that appear in many articles and texts; they describe the fractures as being horizontal.

The second item concerns the fact that the advancing chisel will rotate as the region of the prelacrimal groove is approached. If the handle of the instrument is depressed toward the face and its cutting edge directed slightly medialward at this time, there is a strong probability that it will produce the oblique fracture previously discussed. To ensure this, the instrument can be used as a lever to displace the entire lateral wall medialward.

The third concerns management of convexity of the lateral nasal walls. Laboratory studies indicate that lateral osteotomies performed with chisels often produce hairline fractures that are directed perpendicular to the direction of the cuts. This phenomenon can be used to advantage. Deliberately moving the instrument to and fro after each tap of the mallet will increase the number of perpendicular fractures and make it easy for the surgeon to manipulate the bones with his fingers until multiple additional fractures are produced; this "irons out" the convexity.

Finally, some years ago we described how narrowing can be facilitated by curving the lateral osteotomies upward toward the under surface of the radix when the osteotomy reached the prelacrimal part of the groove (Fig. 104). We called this a "high" osteotomy to distinguish it from the usual osteotomy directed along the prelacrimal groove. Its purpose was to shorten the length of bone that had to be fractured between the upper ends of the medial and lateral osteotomies. It does accomplish that and is particularly useful when the nose is narrow before operation. However, achieving symmetry can become difficult, and, sometimes, the technique produces irregularities when the nose is wide.

CEPHALIC FRACTURE

Some term this "the transverse osteotomy," a misnomer in our opinion because it is not a cut produced with a cutting instrument nor is its direction transverse, if properly performed. Nevertheless, if the medial and lateral osteotomies have been properly performed and if the septum underlying the nasal pyramid is straight and not thickened, producing the obliquely directed cephalic fracture is not difficult. As we have seen, it is brought about by medially directed pressure on the lateral bony walls, the solid radix being used as a fulcrum.

If completion of the cephalic fracture proves difficult, two measures may be helpful (Fig. 105). The blunt blade of a Quisling shatter-fracture osteotome can be introduced beneath the skin and positioned just below the proposed fracture line; tapping the instrument sharply, but firmly, with a mallet will produce the desired fracture. Also, multiple cuts can be made through bone, ice pick fashion, with a 2 or 3 mm osteotome that is introduced through a stab incision in the skin overlying the proposed fracture line; this will facilitate fracture. The incision, made perpendicular to the dorsum, is closed with a fine black silk twist and becomes virtually imperceptible after it heals.

Some surgeons resort to outfracture when infracture of the bones proves difficult. It is not recommended because it may lead to asymmetries, undesirable spicule formation, or the production of a "rocker."

ON COMPLETING THE NARROWING PROCESS

After the cephalic fractures are produced, the bones must be made to touch the septum. This can be accomplished by carefully rasping the medial ends of the fracture lines with an upward-cutting Maltz rasp. If the lower ends of the intact subglabellar segment project unduly, they are, likewise, leveled with the rasp or with a dental drill.

If the nasal dorsum was wide and flat preoperatively, medial osteotomies must be made somewhat lateral to their usual site (Fig. 106). This leaves a widened septal dorsum that must be narrowed later.

The upper lateral cartilages must be considered when narrowing the nose. The cephalic ends extending beneath the nasal bones may remain continuous with the septum when the bony hump is removed (Fig. 107), particularly when it is a small one. When divided later, their medial ends may be in excess and, unless excised, can prevent the bones from satisfactorily approximating the septum.

Another concern is the attachment of the mucous membrane to the medial ends of the upper lateral cartilages, especially in saddle noses. The caudal half of these cartilages is often flattened medially, causing the supratip area to appear wide. This condition can be corrected by dissecting the mucosa from the undersurface of the cartilages so that they can assume their normal configuration when the nose is narrowed.

Finally, the condition known as "returning" of the caudal ends of the upper lateral cartilages may cause the nose to appear widened in the lateral infratip areas; this is easily corrected by excising the bent cartilage (Fig. 108).

Figure 95. Condition of the nasal dorsum after hump removal (right). This is popularly known as an "open roof." The condition must be corrected by mobilizing the lateral walls of the pyramid and moving them medialward so that they meet the septum again.

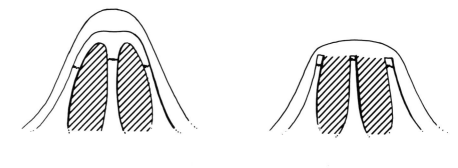

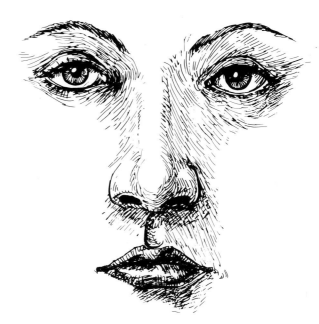

Figure 96. Artistically, the reconstructed nasal dorsum should be about one-half as wide as the intercanthal distance and the nasofacial angles should never lie beyond lines dropped perpendicularly downward from the canthi.

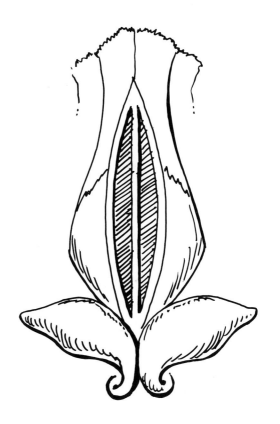

Figure 97. Removal of a bony hump partially separates the nasal bones from each other and from the nasal septum. The length of the separation determines the length of the medial osteotomies subsequently needed.

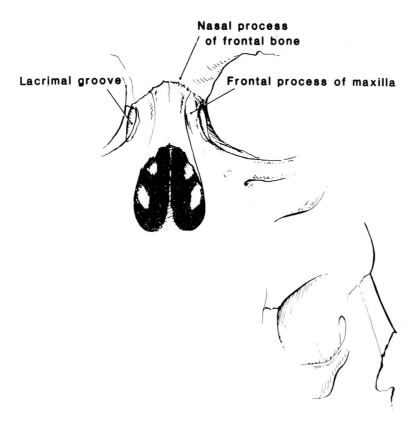

Nasal process of frontal bone

Lacrimal groove

Frontal process of maxilla

Figure 98. The radix nasi is the most solid portion of the external nose. It consists of the nasal process of the frontal bone, the dense upper ends of the nasal bones that overlay and surround the frontal spine, and the frontal processes of the maxillae. Medial osteotomies should never invade the radix.

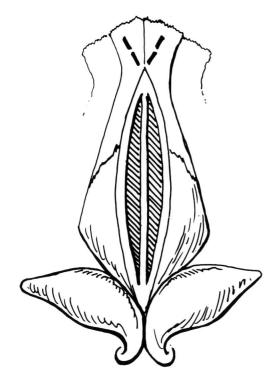

Figure 99. Usual direction of the medial osteotomies. They should veer lateralward as they follow the roof of each nasal vault, and they should never enter the body of the radix nasi.

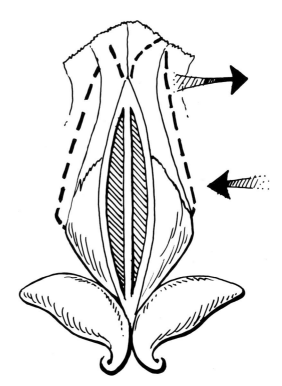

Figure 100. "Rocker" formation. When the medial osteotomy incorrectly enters the body of the radix (left), a fracture of the lateral part of that structure ensues. Since the entire lateral wall of the pyramid remains continuous, narrowing of its lower part causes the upper part of the fractured radix to protrude because the lateral nasal wall "rocks" on a fulcrum formed by the lower part of the body of the radix.

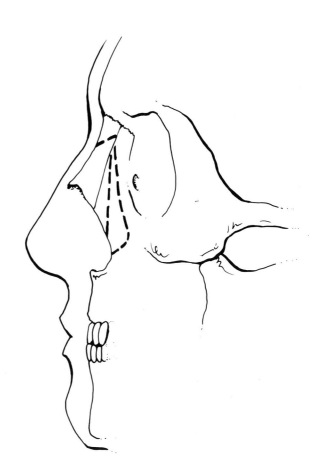

Figure 101. Double osteotomies are performed when the base of the bony pyramid extends beyond the intercanthal boundries. The upper cut determines the new width of the base; the lower one is directed along the existing nasofacial groove.

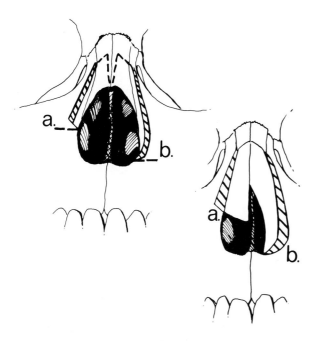

Figure 102. Lateral osteotomies should be started at the level of the anterior ends of the inferior turbinates (a), not lower down along the piriform margins (b); otherwise, the medially displaced lateral walls of the pyramid will block the nasal airway.

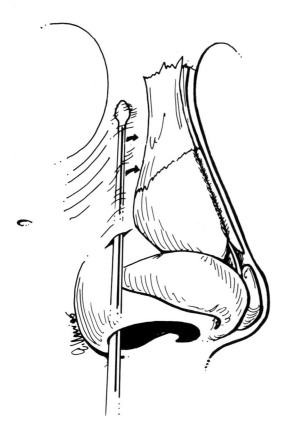

Figure 103. Periosteal tunnels created on both sides of the nasofacial grooves before insertion of the lateral osteotome. An incision is made along the piriform margin at the level of the anterior end of the inferior turbinate. The external tunnel extends into the prelacrimal groove; the internal one extends upward two-thirds as far.

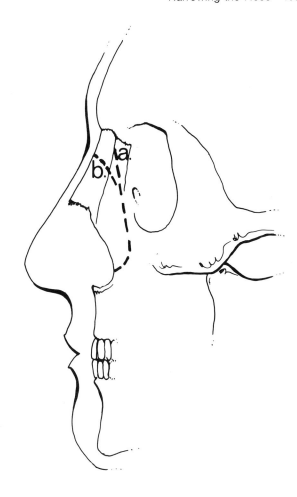

Figure 104. Low and high osteotomies. The low osteotomy (a) is directed along the prelacrimal groove; the high osteotomy (b) is curved toward the nasofrontal angle. The transverse fracture necessary to narrow the nose is shorter when a high osteotomy is performed.

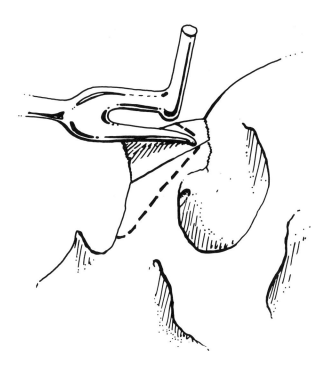

Figure 105. A cephalic fracture that is difficult to produce can be successfully completed with little difficulty if a Quisling shatter-fracture osteotome is used after the inside of the nose has been lightly packed to absorb the force of the blow.

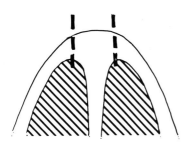

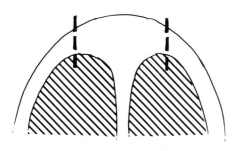

Figure 106. Medial osteotomies should be made further from the midline when the bony dorsum is wide (above); the wideness is then reduced by excising bone from the central segment. This is not necessary when the bony dorsum is narrow.

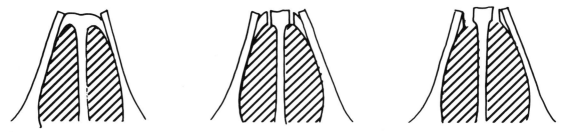

Figure 107. The medial ends of the upper lateral cartilages sometimes remain in excess after bony hump removal and must be excised to permit satisfactory narrowing of the lateral nasal walls.

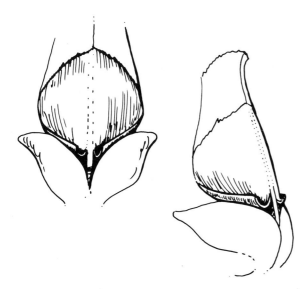

Figure 108. "Returning" of the caudal ends of the upper lateral cartilages that must be excised to narrow the lateral infratip lobule area properly.

15   Postoperative Dressing and Care

After completion of the operative steps, any remaining bony or cartilage debris is extracted from beneath the skin, and bleeding vessels are cauterized with a bipolar cautery, not a difficult task when the external approach is used. WARN-ING: cauterization should be carefully performed to avoid necrosis of the overlying skin.

The skin is then temporarily replaced over the remodeled tip cartilages, and a wet gloved index finger is run along the nasal dorsum to see if there are any residual irregularities that need removal and if the relationship between tip projection and septal dorsum is satisfactory. Next, the transcolumellar and rim incisions are sutured as described in the chapter on nasal base modification.

If septoplasty was performed, the caudal septum is splinted for 1 week between two pieces of exposed x-ray film that have been trimmed so they can be easily introduced and removed through the nostrils and have been notched so that they fit over the piriform margins (Fig. 109). The splints are held in situ with transeptal 4–0 silk sutures.

NASAL DRESSING

We apply a nasal dressing that is left undisturbed for 1 week in all cases; one part splints the bony and cartilagenous pyramid and the other splints the remodeled lobule.

Before the dressing is applied, as much operative edema as possible is reduced by gentle squeezing and finger massage of the nasal covering. Then, the entire nose cephalic to the basal segment is covered with one or two layers of Microform tape that extends from the nasofrontal angle to the supratip depression and lateralward just above the lines of lateral osteotomy (Fig. 110a). This soft, easily removable carpet applies gentle, evenly distributed pressure to the soft tissues overlying the reconstituted nasal skeleton and absorbs pressure generated by postoperative edema. It rarely causes skin irritation, and preliminary use of tincture of benzoin is unnecessary.

We consider the next step to be the most important part of the nasal dressing.

After the uncovered lobule is "milked" of edema once again, it is enclosed with a sling of one-half inch paper tape that does not extend below the nostril apexes; its two ends extend straight upward, parallel to each other and to the nasal dorsum (Fig. 110b). The sling is then apposed to the underlying Microform dressing with a strip of paper tape applied across the supratip area (Fig. 110c). This accomplishes three things: it apposes the supratip soft tissues to the septal dorsum and the columella to the caudal septum and bandages and projects the tip of the nose above the level of the nasal dorsum, usually for a distance of 2 or 3 mm. The tape is crimped around the lobule (Fig. 110c) to produce a neat fit, thereby creating a mold for the remodeled lobular cartilages. The entire area covered by the Microform tape is then covered by overlapping strips of ordinary perforated adhesive tape (Fig. 110d).

Six layers of quick-drying plaster of Paris are cut into a pattern that fits over the perforated tape. After being dipped in hot water, it is molded to the nose with frequently changed surgical sponges until it hardens (Fig. 110e) and produces a strong, yet light, splint that adheres to the remainder of the dressing without the need of additional taping to the surrounding face.

Two pieces of Surgicel of different size are placed into each nostril. The smaller pieces are rolled into small balls and gently inserted into the domes of the vestibule to appose the tip cartilages to the mold; they are left undisturbed until they fall out or can be extracted easily, in from 4 to 7 days. The larger pieces loosely fill the nostrils and are removed the next morning. A small mustache-type dressing made with a 3 by 3 inch gauze wipe is used to catch any leakage.

Worthy of note are the following:

1. The purpose of splinting is to protect the remodeled nose from trauma during the early healing period and to prevent widening of the lateral walls from intranasal edema. In addition, when the continuity of the dorsal septal buttress

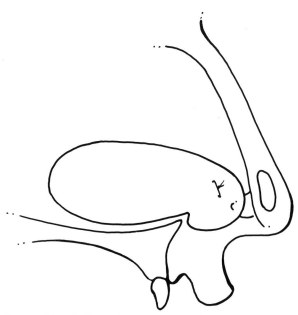

Figure 109. Splints of exposed x-ray film used to support the caudal end of the septum for 1 week after a Metzenbaum swinging door septoplasty. The splints are notched to accomodate the piriform margins and are held in place with a mattress suture of black silk.

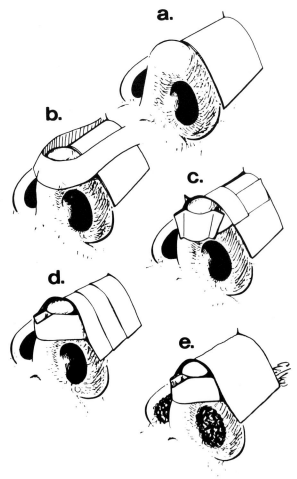

Figure 110. a: One or two layers of Microform tape extending as far as the lines of lateral osteotomy. b: Steri-Strip sling for tip does not extend lower than nostril apexes. c: Arms of sling are taped to Microform, and sling around lobule is crimped. d: All of dressing previously applied is covered with ordinary perforated adhesive tape. e: Plaster of Paris cast is applied over the nasal dorsum. Note that no part of the dressing extends beyond the lines of osteotomy.

has been interrupted as part of concurrent septoplasty, a properly applied dressing splints the septum. However, splinting will not accomplish what has not been done surgically, such as narrow a nose wherein the osteotomies have been imperfect. The surgeon who thinks it will do so is doomed to disappointment.

2. Unless one suspects underlying infection or necrosis, the dressing should not be removed and reapplied during the first postoperative week just for the purpose of inspecting the underlying skin; this will interfere with healing and prolong edema.

3. The dressing should not be extended lateral to the osteotomy lines nor should it be anchored to the remainder of the face with adhesive tape strips because any movement of the muscles of the face will then be transmitted to the nose during the early healing period.

4. It is best not to pack the nasal vestibule before the tip sling is applied because of the distortion it causes and the undue pressure that can be generated during taping. Rather, the sling should be thought of as creating a mold to hold the reconstituted lobular cartilages in the desired position during the early part of healing. The small pieces of Sur-

gicel serve to pack them neatly against the inside of the mold, not to distort them.

5. Packing the nose is not necessary after rhinoplasty, or even septorhinoplasty, if one performs the operation intramucosally, meticulously elevates the membranes, and if the external approach is used so that all bleeding can be visualized and hemostatis established before closure. We believe packing blocks lymph drainage to the nasopharynx, thereby increasing morbidity after operation. There has been no increase in the incidence of postoperative hemorrhage or septal hematoma since we began the practice about 20 years ago.

POSTOPERATIVE CARE

When the patient is returned to his room after surgery, the head of the bed is elevated to a 45° angle and continuous application of cold compresses over the nose and eyes is begun. Mild analgesia, sedation, and antiemetic medication are ordered for use, if necessary. The mustache dressings are changed whenever they become soaked with drippings.

Part of the vestibular packing is removed the next morning, and the patient is discharged with instructions to remain up and about thereafter and to continue the cold compresses for the first 24 hours. A soft diet and moderation in activity are recommended. Also, we prescribe sedation to be used for sleeping difficulty and mild, over-the-counter analgesics to augment the effect of the cold compresses; we recommend against the use of narcotics, if possible, because the grogginess they produce seem to prolong convalescence both physically and psychologically; however, it must be admitted that some patients appear to have a lower pain threshold than others, and they will require stronger medication.

Three days later the transcolumellar and any other external sutures are removed, the base of the nose is cleaned and the patient's progress is monitored. A dose of reassurance is usually necessary. The patient is urged to keep the remainder of the face clean and female patients are taught to cover the circumorbital ecchymosis, if any, with cosmetics.

One week after operation, the external dressing and any remaining synthetic sutures in the nostril areas are removed; the one exception is the septocolumellar "gathering" suture used to narrow the base of the columella. The x-ray film used to splint the caudal end of the septum after septoplasty is removed at this time. Intranasal edema, plus normal bony healing, tends to cause widening of the nose after rhinoplasty, so we demonstrate to most patients a method of manual narrowing (Fig. 111) that we recommend they use for 1 minute at a time 10 to 12 times a day; at first, they are somewhat fearful of the procedure and a little bit tentative in carrying it out, but they soon become quite proficient. This "exercise," as patients want to call it, is continued for 2 or 3 weeks, or until no further movement of the bones can be discerned.

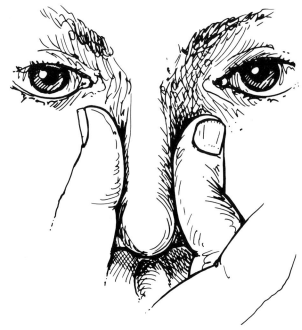

Figure 111. Method of narrowing the nose for 2 or 3 weeks after operation. Object is to overcome widening caused by edema.

The next visit is scheduled 3 or 4 days later to clean the nose, check the progress of healing, determine if the patient has been narrowing the nose properly, and to reassure them about concerns they invariably have.

Three weeks after operation the septocolumellar "gathering" suture is removed and progress is rechecked.

Return visits are scheduled on about 4 or 5 occasions during the ensuing year if the patient is cooperative. We advise them that small intranasal adhesions sometimes occur and should be treated early. Also, we use these visits to inject small amounts (0.1 ml) of triamcinotone acetonide (10 mg/ml) into the supratip area if swelling does not seem to be subsiding quickly enough. In truth, these visits are more desired by us than by the majority of patients; we urge them so that we can see the results of the technical variations used from time to time; in this connection, each patient is sent a recall letter 1 year after the operation for this purpose, but we invite some patients to return even later because the subsidence of operative edema sometimes takes several years, especially in thick-skinned people.

16   Complications

A complication is a condition or state beyond the control of the surgeon that occurs during or after an operation but not as a logical or expected consequence of it.

When performing rhinoplasty, a surgeon is undertaking one of the most complex operations in plastic surgery. As proof, on one occasion we hired a photographer to document every step of a moderately difficult septorhinoplasty and ended up with 134 slides. Additionally, not only must all of the elements fit together like the pieces of a jigsaw puzzle, but the whole must heal properly, not an unimportant factor when one considers that changes secondary to healing may continue in an operated nose for several years.

The range of complications that can occur during or after any operation is truly awesome, so we will consider only those we have found to be the most frequent. They represent inherent risks that the patient must assume if he wants the operation.

EDEMA AND ECCHYMOSIS

Almost every patient develops some facial edema and periorbital ecchymosis after rhinoplasty, even though the operation has been as surgically atraumatic as a human can make it; why people react so differently to trauma is not yet clear.

Aside from a natural desire to make their patients comfortable, surgeons should remember that postoperative edema and ecchymosis "turns off" more prospective patients than anything else; therefore it behooves them to do everything possible to minimize their development.

Things that seem to contribute to postoperative swelling and periorbital ecchymosis after operation include lengthy operating time, difficulties encountered during osteotomies, performing concomitant submucous resection or septoplasty, and agitation, hypertension, and vomiting during or immediately after the procedure.

We attempt to minimize their development in several ways:

1. Citrobioflavonoids are prescribed for several days before the operation. Parenthetically, we have noted that patients who routinely take sustained-release vitamin C daily seem to do better than those who do not. The same is true of those who exercise regularly or might be considered "vitamin freaks."
2. The patient is adequately sedated before and during operation.
3. Intravenous Permarin 20 mg is administered to patients who are postmenopausal and to those who are or have just concluded menstruating.
4. A studied attempt is made to avoid the angular and infraorbital vessels during local anesthetic infiltration. In addition, the operation is not started until vasoconstriction is well established.
5. The blood pressure is closely monitored during operation, and lowering measures are instituted immediately if elevation begins.
6. The airway is constantly monitored to guard against an increase in carbon dioxide and the vasodilation it can cause.
7. The procedure is performed expeditiously so the time frame of vasoconstrictor effectiveness is not exceeded.
8. The operation is performed intramucosally in an attempt to minimize operative and postoperative hemorrhage.
9. Bleeding vessels encountered during the surgery are immediately controlled with bipolar coagulation.
10. The traumatic part of the operation, that is, the osteotomies, are not performed until the end of the procedure so that the postoperative dressing can be applied as soon as possible thereafter.
11. Dexamethasone 10 mg is administered intravenously just before osteotomies are performed in the hope of reducing edema.

12. Nasal packing is not used even though septal surgery has been done, because, as noted previously, we believe it contributes to facial edema by blocking lymph drainage to the nasopharynx. This is made possible by meticulous elevation and hemostasis during submucous resection or septoplasty. We do splint the caudal septum with exposed x-ray film for 1 week after septoplasty to immobilize the caudal septum, not for hemostasis.

13. The nasal dressing is confined to the nose, not anchored to the face with strips of adhesive tape that transmit facial movements to the healing nose.

14. When the patient is returned to her room, the head of the bed is elevated to a 45° angle and continuous cold compresses are applied over the nose and surrounding face until the following morning. The blood pressure is also monitored, and the mustache dressing is left largely undisturbed unless there is excessive leakage.

15. The patient is advised to remain out of bed after returning home, to avoid any activity that might elevate the blood pressure, and to continue the cold compresses for 24 hours, albeit at a reduced rate.

The minimal swelling and discoloration that most patients experience has almost disappeared after 7 to 10 days. The small amount of edema remaining takes a year or more to subside, and we have encountered some instances wherein small amounts of iron pigment remained in the skin for several years before disappearing.

HEMORRHAGE

Hemorrhage requiring intervention after surgery is rare in our experience, even though we do some type of septal repair at the time of rhinoplasty approximately 95 percent of the time. Perhaps, performing the operation intramucosally and via the external approach permits better intraoperative hemostasis than would be possible otherwise.

If bleeding does occur, the source is usually found in one of the lateral osteotomy incisions, and it can be controlled by silver nitrate cauterization followed by packing with Surgicel.

When bleeding arises from lacerations of the septal membrane or the mucosa underlying the lateral osteotomies, an attempt is made to locate the bleeding point after shrinking the tissues with a vosoconstrictor; it is then cauterized and the nose is packed with Surgicel. If sufficient compression is not obtained by this means, the nose is packed with 1 inch roll gauze that has been impregnated with petrolatum. This packing is left undisturbed for 48 hours and then removed piecemeal during the next 2 or 3 days. Of course, whenever packing of this nature is used, antibiotic coverage is indicated.

A septal hematoma is generally recognizable, but a no. 16 needle should be introduced for aspiration of any suspicious swelling of the septum. If a hematoma is found, it should be aspirated daily until bloody return is no longer obtained; repacking is not necessary after aspiration. Virtually painless needling can be accomplished by, first, anesthetizing the mucosa with a cotton pledget that has been soaked in a solution of 2% tetracaine and, later, injecting 2% lidocaine containing 1:100,000 epinephrine directly into the membrane. Antibiotic prophylaxis is always indicated against the development of a septal abscess.

SKIN COMPLICATIONS

Small pustules are sometimes found when the tape dressing is removed; they are usually of no moment and do not recur after being ruptured during skin cleaning.

Increased pilosebaceous activity for a short time frequently occurs after rhinoplasty; it can be particularly annoying in people with oily skin and in those who are timid about touching the nose after operation. The most effective treatment consists of cleansing the nose several times daily with a good soap (we recommend Neutrogena), until the condition subsides; if this is not done, a thin, rough coagulum that blocks the pores and, thereby, perpetuates the swelling will form. It may even be necessary to dissolve the film with a skin cleanser, such as Sebanil.

SKIN NECROSIS

Necrosis of the skin is very rare but can occur as a result of injudicious use of the electrocautery on its undersurface or from a dressing that is applied too tightly or becomes too tight after postoperative swelling occurs. Of course, one should be careful when using cautery on the undersurface of the skin; a wet-field bipolar cautery whose tips have been dipped in water is recommended because hemostasis can sometimes be achieved simply by holding the wet tips close to the bleeding vessel.

The tip sling portion of the nasal dressing should never extend below the nostril apexes and should be divided whenever the columella and tip appears inflamed or swollen or the patient complains of throbbing pain in the area.

Once established, necrosis should be treated the same as it is treated anywhere else, that is, by debridement, encouragement of granulation, watchful waiting, attempts to modify scar contracture with intralesional triamcinolone acetonide (10 mg/ml) after several weeks have passed, and, later, reconstruction.

INFECTION

Fortunately, infection after rhinoplasty or septorhinoplasty is rare, probably because it is generally conceded that one should not operate on a patient who gives a history of an active or recent upper respiratory or skin infection and because of the widespread use of prophylactic antibiotics.

However, infection can occur as a result of hematoma formation or around bone dust or fragments, especially when there is an avenue open to the surface of the nasal mucosa. Using bank cartilage without prior removal of all of its perichondrium causes a rejection phenomenon that resembles infection.

Of all surgical specialists, otolaryngologists would seen to be best equipped by training to diagnose and treat nasal infections.

NASAL BLOCKAGE

Some patients complain of prolonged nasal obstruction after rhinoplasty even though intranasal examination reveals no residual structural abnormality. When allergy and failure to clear accumulated crusts from the nose by blowing is ruled out, we are left with a few people in whom the neuromuscular control of the vessels in the nasal mucosa is apparently disturbed by the operation. Fortunately, the condition usually clears spontaneously as time passes, but the patient needs reassurance in the interim and should be warned against resorting to the use of nose drops. On rare occasions, submucous resection of the inferior turbinates may be in order; incidentally, competent rhinologists shun the practice of almost routine turbinectomy that is advocated in some circles today.

SEPTAL PERFORATION

It is impossible for a surgeon not to lacerate the mucosa when correcting some severe septal deformities, particularly those produced by one or more traumatic episodes. Unilateral lacerations, large or small, are usually not of great concern, because membrane regeneration will close them without incident. However, opposing bilateral tears will result in permanent septal perforation unless each side is repaired separately with sutures and a piece of septal cartilage or temporalis fascia is sandwiched between the flaps.

EXCESSIVE PATIENT DEPENDENCE

Despite seemingly flawless preparation, a few patients do not cope well with the rigors of the undertaking, seem to enjoy ill-health, as it were, and require repeated reassurance that, for instance, their swelling will eventually subside, that their sense of smell and taste will return, that tip projection will decrease, that smiling will again become facile, and so on. Fortunately, they constitute a very small segment of the rhinoplasty population, and a good office assistant can be trained to handle judiciously the majority of their telephone calls and the minor complaints they seem to dwell on. The condition usually subsides spontaneously with the passage of time, but the good humor of the surgeon and his staff can be sorely taxed in the meantime.

17   Secondary Rhinoplasty

When one considers the complexity and psychologic overtones of the operation, the widely varying expertise of surgeons, and the infinite variety of deformities they encounter, it is a wonder that most rhinoplasties turn out as successful as they do.

One reason may be that the criterion for success in rhinoplasty is patient satisfaction, not surgeon satisfaction. Fortunately, most patients are realistic and seek improvement, not perfection. Nevertheless, a small number do request revision either from their own surgeon or from some other surgeon; sometimes their request is justified, sometimes not. On occasion, it is the operating surgeon who suggests revision because he feels additional improvement is possible.

If rhinoplasty is a complex operation, revision rhinoplasty can be even more complex, so it should not be undertaken lightly. Whether correcting his own work or that of others, the surgeon must work in a scarred, already altered environment that makes results less predictable and more likely to fall short of expectations. Furthermore, he is often dealing with a disappointed, possibly disaffected patient who, secretly, still hopes to reach the goal of his original undertaking. Thus, in addition to special technical problems, secondary rhinoplasty often has unique ethical, psychologic, and medicolegal overtones that can make even the most experienced surgeon hesitant.

WHAT IS A SATISFACTORY RESULT?

It has been said, and rightly so, that the object of cosmetic rhinoplasty is improvement, not perfection. This implies that the surgeon has achieved a degree of improvement that would be considered acceptable to qualified observers in view of the type of nose originally presented by the patient and the state of the art.

There was no objective method of studying improvement until we began using a scale based on photographic analysis of the nose before operation (Fig. 112). Every defect in the nose is assigned a value, and the total is subtracted from 100 to establish the preoperative grade given to the nose. The process is repeated 1 year after operation to determine how much improvement the surgery accomplished.

Our experience has been that it should be possible to improve the average nontraumatized, developmental deformity without thickened skin by about 20 to 30 points. Less improvement should be anticipated in revision rhinoplasty, as a rule. Therefore, a satisfactory result would be one wherein most of the preoperative defects had been eliminated and some of those remaining represent improvement. Conversely, an unsatisfactory result would be one wherein there remains gross evidence of deformity or deranged function; certainly, the postoperative grade of the nose should never be worse than the preoperative one unless some complication occurred.

CAUSES OF UNSATISFACTORY RESULTS

Unsatisfactory results may stem from operative complications or sequelae. We have already noted that a complication is a condition or state that occurs during or after operation, but not as a logical or expected consequence of it.

Sequelae, on the other hand, follow as a logical consequence of what is done or not done during operation, or they might result from poor selection and preparation of patients or uninspired planning. If surgical execution is faulty, the error may be in judgment, ommission, or commission.

Most secondary deformities are sequelae of the operation, not complications. That is why most articles on secondary rhinoplasty emphasize prevention and warn inexperienced surgeons to tread lightly in the area of revision operations. Parenthetically, this emphasizes the need to study constantly one's results in an objective manner so that recurrent technical deficiencies can be noted and eliminated.

RHINOPLASTY SCALE

NAME _____ Surgery date ___/___/___ Date p.o. study ___/___/___

FRONTAL VIEW	Pre	Post
NASAL DORSUM		
Deviation from midline		
Bony portion (2)		
Cartilagenous portion (2)		
Width		
Radix area (2)		
Bony portion (2)		
Cartilagenous portion (2)		
Depressions		
Bony portion (1)		
Cartilagenous portion (1)		
NASAL BASE		
Width of lobule (2)		
Width of alae (2)		
Alar flare (2)		
Deviation of lobule (2)		
Inequality alar levels (1)		
Alar cartilages		
Depressions (1)		
Discrete prominences (1)		
Skin quality (1)		
LATERAL NASAL WALLS		
Width at nasofacial angles		
Upper third (2)		
Middle third (2)		
Lower third (alae not included) (2)		
Depressions		
Nasal bones (R - L) (1)		
U.L. cartilages (R - L) (1)		
Prominences		
Nasal bones (R - L) (1)		
U.L. cartilages (R - L) (1)		

LATERAL VIEW	Pre	Post
NASAL DORSUM		
Nasofrontal angle depth (2)		
Nasal dorsum (not lobule)		
Convexity		
Bony portion (2)		
Cartilagenous portion (2)		
Soft tissue (1)		
Concavity		
Bony portion (2)		
Cartilagenous portion (2)		
Absence supratip break (1)		
Projection of pyramid		
Excessive (2)		
Deficient (2)		
Length of dorsum (including lobule)		
Excessive (2)		
Deficient (2)		
NASAL BASE		
Tip projection		
Excessive (2)		
Deficient (2)		
Columella		
Hanging (2)		
Retracted (2)		
Columella-lip ratio (1)		
Level disparity medial-lateral crura (1)		
Caudal contour of nose		
Medial crura angulation (1)		
Too straight (1)		
Webbing nasolabial angle (1)		
Notching of alae (1)		
Length facial plane of pyramid (2)		

BASAL VIEW

LOBULE	Pre	Post
Height (2)		
Configuration (triangle) (2)		
Dome assymetries (2)		
Bifidity (2)		
Knuckling (2)		
NOSTRILS		
Shape (2)		
Assymetries (1)		
Long axes (2)		
Double sill (1)		

PRE-OP SCORE: _____ POST-OP SCORE: _____

COLUMELLA	Pre	Post
Length (1)		
Lobule height/length ratio (1)		
Deviation (2)		
Caudal septal distortion (2)		
Splayed crural feet		
Unilateral (1)		
Bilateral (1)		
Widening base (2)		
Bifidity (1)		
Scarring (1)		
ALAE		
Thickened (1)		
Poor scarring (1)		

© Jack R. Anderson M.D.

Figure 112.   Rhinoplasty scale used to grade noses before and after operation.

REVISIONAL SURGERY GUIDELINES

Certain principles might be recommended as guidelines regarding revisional surgery.

1. It is doubtful if one should suggest revision when the patient is satisfied with the result of the original operation. The surgeon who does so is assuming that he can make the patient even more satisfied than satisfied, a delicate and dangerous undertaking.

2. If one's own patient requests correction of an obvious deformity that can be remedied without too much downside risk, they should be reoperated on, but only 9 to 12 months after the original operation; by that time, most of the tissue changes resulting from the first intervention will have subsided.

3. No one should be accepted for reoperation unless there is gross evidence of deformity or deranged function. The fact that the original surgery did not quite accomplish what the patient had intended should not be the determining factor. Surgeons should remember several things: people who request correction of minor residual deformities are patently more critical and demanding than the average; precise surgery becomes more difficult in a scarred environment; the percentage of improvement possible is smaller; the downside risk is greater; and the time must be propitious. Finally, it should be recalled: "The enemy of good is better."

4. When the original surgery was done elsewhere, it is wise to be noncommittal and diplomatic when patients try to fix blame for their predicament, as many are wont to do. Sometimes, their probing is open and above board, sometimes surreptitious. In truth, a firm opinion as to cause cannot always be formulated, inasmuch as there is no way of knowing what problems were faced by the first surgeon nor what happened during or after the procedure. About all a consultant can tell the patient is what is wrong with the nose and the treatment indicated, if any.

5. Patients being considered for revision of surgery done elsewhere should be subjected to even more stringent psychologic selection than new patients are. Most are only hapless victims of surgical misadventures and respond favorably to a second operation if there is only moderate improvement. However, some are unrealistic, deep-seated, and obstinate perfectionists or appearance neurotics who seem to be expending too much psychic energy on the deformity and are only too willing to undergo numerous operations in pursuit of their illusions. It is well to remember, too, that their disappointment may be superimposed on emotional disturbances that were present before the first operation, so their ability to cope with yet another possible disappointment becomes questionable and could lead to decompensation. Thus, psychiatric consultation seems indicated more often in these people than in the general population of rhinoplasty seekers.

6. Before undertaking secondary rhinoplasty, the surgeons should honestly assess his ability to help the patient by asking himself the following questions and answering them truthfully:
     Do I have enough experience and technical ability to help this patient? If so, how much improvement can I achieve, and will it be enough to satisfy him?
     Will the condition be worsened if the intervention is unsuccessful?
     Would the patient and my career be better served by referring him to someone who is more experienced?
   Operating beyond one's competence is not only a disservice, but usually spawns inferior results. It can be particularly disastrous in this type of surgery wherein the results of one's efforts are like a traveling billboard for all to see, wherein success depends on patient rather than doctor satisfaction, and wherein so much of the patient's contentment depends on the validation he or she receives from others. All things considered, young surgeons should be superselective in choosing patients for secondary operations; the desire to operate, for whatever reason, and any "rescue complex" he may have should be subverted.

7. Before accepting a patient for secondary

operation, a thorough history should be taken and physical examination performed and photographic analysis made.

8. The happiest results of revision surgery are usually attained when the first operation was not completed as, for example, when a cartilagenous polly beak deformity results from insufficient lowering of the cartilagenous septal dorsum. Correction becomes more difficult after excessive or unskilled surgery, when there is an excessive accumulation of scar tissue, or when there is tissue deficit. Likewise, results of postoperative infection are usually difficult to correct. Finally, it should be recognized that some noses are beyond redemption; the case of a woman who had undergone 28 previous nasal operations is a case in point.

9. Except when only minor corrections are indicated, revision rhinoplasty is usually best done via the open approach. Exposure is superb. Working room is unmatched. The surgeon can see the causes of disfigurement and tell immediately how effective his corrective efforts have been. Subcutaneous accumulations of scar tissue can be precisely eliminated without too much difficulty, thereby allowing the nasal covering to be returned to almost its original degree of pliancy. Structures that are bound down or distorted by scar tissue can be released more easily and completely. Implants can be placed and secured into position with exactness.

10. Fundamentals of revision surgery include:

It is essential to restore the pliability of the covering of the pyramid in most cases.

Structures distorted by scar tissue contracture must be mobilized.

The operation should be done by the open method and intramucosally, if possible.

Tissue implants, not synthetics, should be used for augmentation or replacement, if possible.

Complete whatever was not done at the first operation.

Do not depend on splints or sutures to accomplish the goals of the correction.

SPECIFIC DEFORMITIES

An infinite variety of secondary deformities have been encountered in the postrhinoplasty population; some can be treated successfully, others cannot.

Only a number of the more common ones can be discussed here.

Polly Beak Deformities

Two types are recognized, one caused by postoperative accumulation of soft tissue in the supratip area, and the other by insufficient lowering of the skeletal elements, particularly the septal dorsum.

Soft tissue polly beaks can usually be prevented at the time of surgery by excising excessive supratip subcutaneous tissue so that the skin drapes properly and by lengthening the medial crura with a cartilagenous strut so that the tip does not "drop" after operation; it must be admitted, however, that there are instances wherein thickened skin subverts one's best efforts.

When development is detected early, the condition often responds to several biweekly injections of 0.02 ml of triamcinolone (10 mg/ml) directly into the area beginning 3 or 4 weeks after operation. If this treatment is unsuccessful, excision of the entire sheet of scar tissue, plus careful crosshatching of the undersurface of the dermis is done 9 to 12 months later; additional trimming of the septal dorsum, upper lateral or lobular cartilages, or augmentation of tip support may also be necessary. However, lowering of the projection of the septal dorsum alone will not correct a soft tissue polly beak; it will only lead to the formation of more hypertrophic scar tissue.

A warning: triamcinolone should not be used earlier than 3 or 4 weeks after operation, nor should the 40 mg/ml formulation ever be used because it can cause subcutaneous atrophy that might require several months for reversal.

A cartilagenous polly beak deformity results from failure to secondarily lower the projection of the septal dorsum and the upper lateral cartilages at the end of rhinoplasty. Correction is not difficult and consists of completing the operation.

Scarring of the Skin

Scars may result from accidental perforation of the skin during operation, infection, or necrosis.

A combination of sharp and blunt dissection

with curved iris scissors is usually safer than scalpel dissection when undermining the skin in secondary operations; the tips of the scissors should be pointed in the direction of the nasal skeleton because the probability of skin perforation is especially high, and often unavoidable, in secondary corrections wherein the skeletal structures are tightly bound down by scar tissue.

When the skin is lacerated during dissection, the margins of the wound should be carefully approximated with 6–0 or 7–0 suture "twists" that can be removed in 3 or 4 days to avoid leaving suture scars; the wound margins are then supported for an additional period of time with strips of paper adhesive tape. If the scar begins to thicken, intralesional injections of triamcinolone (10 mg/ml) can be used on several occasions to improve its appearance, and wire-brush dermabrasion of the scar at the end of 6 weeks frequently does wonders.

Large scars may result from skin necrosis secondary to cauterization of bleeding vessels on the undersurface of the skin, infection, or pressure from the bandage.

Bleeding vessels on the undersurface of the skin should be cauterized gingerly, if at all, with a wet-field bipolar cautery. The dressing should be removed at the first hint of skin infection beneath the bandage, and the adhesive tape sling around the lobule should not be applied too tightly, should not extend onto the columella, and should be released if there is a great deal of postoperative swelling from whatever reason.

Once necrosis is established, little can be done until reepithelialization of the depressed area is complete. This occurs rapidly when the area is small, but large areas may require debridement and the application of Scarlet Red or Dermaid, an aloe preparation useful in full-thickness burn treatment, to speed the process. Later, dermabrasion of the edges of the scar might be tried to cause them to blend in with the surrounding skin. After 9 to 12 months have passed, the scar can be excised and the deficit repaired with flaps or a full-thickness skin graft obtained from the postauricular region.

"Dimpling" of the Skin

This condition arises when the undersurface of the skin heals directly to mucosa because there is no intervening cartilage or bone. Thus, it may occur when there is an open roof, that is, when the nasal bones do not abut the septum after osteotomies. A variant is the pinched tip caused by internal scar contracture plus excessive removal of upper and lower lateral cartilages.

Performing the operation intramucosally, properly executing narrowing, and maintaining the skeletal continuity of the cartilages will prevent the condition.

Once established, it can be corrected by elevating the skin, dividing the scar, and interposing a thin layer of crushed cartilage to prevent its reformation; the open roof should be closed, if present.

Skeletal Irregularities

Postoperative irregularities visible or palpable beneath the skin of the nose have many causes: imprecise skeletal trimming and smoothing; retention of fragments of bones or cartilages; irregular bony infracture during lateral osteotomy; performing lateral osteotomy at too high a level, thereby creating the so-called stair-step deformity; failure to level the uppermost part of the nasal hump or any projection of the "K" (keystone) area; failure to correct "returning" of the caudal ends of the upper lateral cartilages; bending or elevation of cartilage caused by scar contracture during healing; and, finally, thinness of the skin that causes even minute irregularities to be visible.

As always, the best treatment is prevention. Inspection of the exposed nasal framework at the end of operation might reveal potential problems. "Sweeping" the area and the undersurface of the overlying skin with a medium Maltz rasp usually removes fragments of bone and cartilage. Wetting a gloved finger improves tactile sensitivity when it is passed along the dorsum to search for small irregularities, especially after both nostrils have been depressed toward the premaxillae to throw the dorsum into relief.

When the skin is thin, we have found two measures useful: placing a layer of Gelfoam along the entire length of the nasal dorsum or doing the same with a thin layer of crushed cartilage. If the cut ends of the lower lateral cartilages are evident through the skin at the end of operation, they should be trimmed or morselized; they, too, can be covered with a thin layer of crushed cartilage.

A palpable ledge of bone visible at the lower end of the radix may result when the infraradix fracture lines occur at different levels when the nose is narrowed or, perhaps, when one nasal wall was moved medially further than the other. Removing any obstacle to equalize medial movement will correct the condition; if this is unsuccessful, the overhang may be leveled with an upward cutting Maltz rasp or removed with a narrow Lempert rongeur.

Performing a lateral osteotomy too far above the nasofacial groove will create a so-called stair-step deformity, so it behooves one to palpate the levels of the lateral osteotomies before concluding the operation and performing a second osteotomy at a lower level, if necessary.

Special mention should be made of the residual "humps" that are frequently seen after operations performed by, even, the best surgeons; they are often dismissed summarily with such statements as, "I like a small hump of a nose after operation; it makes it look natural." That is a cop-out, it seems to us, because a hump is a hump is a hump, and it would be better if it were not there, even though the nose has been vastly improved by operation and the patient has been given advance notice that the result will not be perfect.

Residual dorsal convexities, aside from polly break deformities, usually occur at two places, where the original bony hump begins cephalically and at the "K" area, where the septal dorsum dips under the caudal end of the bony dorsum. They should be searched for assiduously at the end of operation and corrected if found. Slight projections caused by the residual cephalic end of the hump are often difficult to discern, unless one is performing open rhinoplasty, because their presence is frequently masked by the overlying procerus muscle. The medial ends of the upper lateral cartilages in the "K" area require special attention because they often bend inward when cut from the septum, and they can interfere with reforming the roof of the pyramid.

"Bossing" of the tip is another irregularity that deserves being highlighted. It refers to projections that sometimes appear as long as a year or two after rhinoplasty when the complete strip technique of lobular modification is used inappropriately, that is, when the upper ends of the medial crura are twisted or bent, an indication that abnormal developmental tensions are locked in those cartilages. True "bossing" will not occur when the lower lateral cartilages are divided at their angles and part of the medial ends of each lateral crus is excised to relieve the tension that, otherwise, will be intensified unpredictably by scar tissue contracture during healing.

Secondary correction is accomplished in the same manner as if the irregularities were discovered at the end of operation, that is, by excision and completing the procedure, if necessary; however, exposure and freeing the tangled structures from scar tissue is, often, very difficult. Finally, it becomes virtually impossible to correct depressions in some instances except with implants or morselized or crushed cartilage.

Saddle Nose Deformity

Saddling may involve the entire dorsum or just the supratip area. Saddling of the entire dorsum can be caused by too much hump removal, displacement of the bony walls into the nose during narrowing, or disruption of the continuity of the dorsal septal buttress after submucous resection, in which case the nose is, also, shortened considerably. Saddling of the supratip area almost invariably follows loss of the caudal portion of the septal cartilage due to infection or hematoma; it may, likewise, result from lowering the projection of the caudal end of the septal dorsum too much.

Excessive hump removal is avoided by determining in advance how much the nasal dorsum should be lowered based on a line joining the nasal tip at its proposed new location and the planned or existing nasofrontal angle.

The bony walls can be displaced downward into the nasal cavity by using excessive force to accomplish infracture. Preserving attachment of the bones to the overlying skin helps to prevent this, so only enough skin to permit instrumentation during hump removal should be elevated from the bony dorsum. Even so, when forcible infracture is necessary, as with the Quisling instrument, it is wise to insert a moderate amount of packing beneath the bones in advance to limit dislocation. Preserving the periosteum during hump removal and the performance of lateral osteotomy also offers a measure of support.

When repairing a saddle nose, the operation should be performed instramucosally so that any implant used is not exposed to the interior of the nose. Additionally, the upper lateral cartilages should be separated from the septum and a few millimeters of the underlying mucosa is dissected from their medial borders to correct their usual curved configuration. We prefer to use autogenous septal or auricular cartilage implants to correct saddle deformities; if it is not available, banked septal cartilage may be used, but only after meticulously removing any attached mucoperichondrium. In either case, the septal cartilage is morselized or crushed so that it conforms to the shape of the dorsum that has been previously smoothed to eliminate irregularities. The implants should be long enough to fill the entire concavity rather than using several placed in tandem. They may be layered, particularly in the supratip area, to achieve the desired thickness; when this is done, the pieces are sewn together with catgut suture and one or two thicknesses of Supramid mesh is sandwiched between the grafts to enhance tissue fluid perfusion. Ear cartilage cannot be morselized as well as septal cartilage because it tends to fragment, but it can be softened if one is careful.

Implant insertion should be deferred until the very end of operation, just before the dressing is applied, to lessen the possibility of displacement.

When saddling is caused by disruption of the dorsal septal buttress during or subsequent to the first operation, the depressed septal cartilage must be elevated after being separated from the upper lateral cartilages and after its mucosa has been elevated bilaterally, including its attachments to the nasal spine, premaxillary alae, and part of the neighboring piriform margins. Such wide detachment permits the lower lateral cartilages to be pulled caudalward before the newly positioned dorsum is sewn to the upper lateral cartilages near the caudal ends of the nasal bones. Transseptal mattress sutures are, also, inserted beneath the divided buttress so that it is supported from below. Even so, dorsal implants usually must be used in addition to these measures.

Supratip saddling usually causes the appearance of a bony pseudohump that frequently requires leveling for esthetic purposes before long dorsal implants can be used, although it might be possible to correct the condition with supratip implants only. In any case, a cartilage implant placed between the medial crura might be necessary to improve tip projection, too.

Shallow Nasofrontal Angle

If a shallow nasofrontal angle is due to a hypertrophied procerus muscle, this residuum can be corrected by removing that muscle. If the problem is bony, the area can be deepened with a chisel or rotating burr after the soft tissues have been widely elevated. It is important to remember that the remainder of the dorsum must, also, be modified to some degree after deepening.

Excessive Shortening

The cause of this sequela is usually overzealous septal shortening and nasal base rotation during the original operation, although it may accompany saddling caused by disruption of the caudal buttress of cartilage after submucous resection or septoplasty.

As previously noted, most of the length of the nasal dorsum is due to the length, direction, and width of the lateral crura, so septal shortening is needed infrequently, provided the lateral crura are managed properly.

We have rarely been successful in lengthening an overly shortened nose except with the technique devised by Walter; this consists of separating the lower cartilagenous vault from the remainder of the nose by transfixion and intercartilagenous incisions, pulling the lower vault caudalward and filling the dehiscence created with a composite graft obtained from the concha. Multiple interventions may be necessary to fine tune the results of this reconstructive procedure; even then, the supratip area may appear somewhat bulky.

Nasolabial Angle Retraction

Excision of too much of the caudal end of the septum, particularly from the area of the inferior septal angle, may cause this condition; It may be corrected, at times, simply by rotation of the lateral crura, but, usually, so-called plumping grafts of cartilage must be inserted into the base of the columella in addition to improve projection of the area.

When the condition is due to excessive scarring behind the base of the columella after excision of septal lining, repair is difficult and generally unsatisfying in our experience; the scar must be resected and tissue brought in to correct the deficit.

Open Roof Syndrome

When one or both bony lamina fail to abut the septal dorsum after operation, the patient is said to have an open roof. The condition is usually due to faulty narrowing, and patients in whom no attempt was made to narrow the nose after hump removal are still occasionally encountered today.

A unilateral open roof commonly arises from failure to complete the cephalic fracture on one side when an attempt is made to infracture one of the bony lamina; the nose appears crooked in such cases. Treatment, obviously, consists of completing the cephalic fracture during the secondary operation.

Stair-Step Deformity

Performing lateral osteotomies too high on the frontal process of the maxillae instead of in the nasofacial grooves produces prominent ridges where the lateral walls of the nose join the face. Treatment consists of performing secondary osteotomies at the proper level.

Deviation of the Nose

Nasal deviation after operation may have a myriad of causes. As mentioned previously, it may stem from failure to complete narrowing of one side, or it may result from neglecting to equalize the laminae of the bony and/or upper cartilagenous vaults, or, even, unmatched lateral crura. Most often, however, the culprit is deviation of the underlying septum or of the frontal or nasal spines.

Whatever the causes, the operation must be completed during secondary rhinoplasty. The technique is the same as that described in Chapter 13, but it is made more difficult by the altered anatomy and the scar tissue resulting from the first operation.

The septum and its adnexae must be exposed and freed from scar tissue, any unfinished work completed, and the lateral walls, both bone and upper lateral cartilages, and mucous membrane must be equalized. The bony walls of the nose must be mobilized once again, and both the pyramid and reconstructed nasal septum splinted for 1 week.

Even when one succeeds in straightening the septum and shifting the nose to the midline, a slight depression of the nasal bones or upper lateral cartilages on one or both sides may persist, so it becomes necessary to correct the sunken area by implantation one or more layers of appropriately trimmed crushed septal cartilage.

One's best efforts sometimes fall short of complete success; therefore patients should be warned of this possibility in advance. If the surgeon did not perform the original operation, he should portray himself as someone who is trying to help but cannot estimate the amount of improvement that is possible.

Lobule Deviation

Although usually caused by deviation of the underlying caudal end of the septal cartilage, deviation of the lobule may present independently as a result of lower lateral cartilage inequality or torsion of the medial crura. The cause becomes evident after the cartilages have been exposed. The lateral crura are made alike, and the medial crura are straightened by morselization or by excision of segments from the bends after they have been

separated; when sections are excised, it is wise to insert an intracrural batten of septal cartilage before they are sewn together again.

Columellar Deviation

Likewise, this condition is usually caused by deviation of the underlying septum but may be caused by twisting of the medial crura; often, a crooked nasal spine that was not corrected during the original operation is at fault.

Treatment consists of straightening the caudal septum and nasal spine or correcting the twisted medial crura, as was described in the last section.

Hanging Columella

The condition is caused by excessive wideness or convexity of the medial crura or may appear secondary to postoperative elevation of the alar margins due to too generous removal of lateral crura followed by scar contracture; rarely is it caused by a cartilagenous septum that is too long, as is commonly held.

Treatment generally consists of exposing the caudal ends of the medial crura and excising the convexity until their curvature is acceptable. When elevation of the alar margins is the cause, an attempt should be made to move the displaced alar cartilages caudalward, but the use of intranasal composite grafts are frequently indicated.

Widened Columellar Base

This condition may be due to excessive soft tissue, to abnormal flaring of the lower ends of the medial crura, or to a combination of both.

In any case, the soft tissue must be cut out, the adjacent skin of the floor of the nostrils and upper lip undermined, if necessary, and the lower part of the columella gathered with a 000 polypropylene stitch left in situ for about 4 weeks. The lower ends of the medial crura may have to be transected, in which case the severed ends are included in the gathering suture.

Alar Widening

When the tip of the nose is allowed to descend toward the premaxillae after rhinoplasty, the alae will flare or widen and usually cause, in the process, a change in the long axes of the nostrils; or the condition may indicate that the nostrils were not narrowed during the original operation. In either event, the conditions can be improved, as a rule, by using the nostril narrowing technique outlined in Chapter 11.

Alar Notching

Displacement of one of the lateral crural flaps after the cartilage delivery technique of lobular reconstruction is one cause of alar notching. It can be prevented by suturing the flaps to the nostril margins at the end of operation, before the dressing is applied. Once established, it can be treated by mobilizing and repositioning the displaced flap.

As previously indicated, the condition can be caused by excessive narrowing of the lateral crura and, then, upward displacement by scar tissue contracture later. In such cases, the crura and the nasal covering must be mobilized before making an attempt to move the displaced crura caudalward. Because the condition is often accompanied by mucosal deficit, the use of composite grafts may be indicated.

Some degree of alar notching is almost routinely seen when the columella has become shortened and the nasal tip has "dropped" following rhinoplasty; it is but a part of a condition we have dubbed "the surgically shortened columella syndrome"; it consists of supratip soft tissue rounding, nasolabial angle retraction, shortening of the columella because the feet of the medial crura descend until they are even with the floor of the nostrils, widening of the alae and, of course, notching of the alae. Prevention consists of conservation treatment of the caudal septum along with support of the tip at the conclusion of the operation. Treatment consists of liberating the lateral crura and increasing the length of the medial crura, if possible, with an intracrural strut of cartilage; the surrounding tissues may have to be mobilized, and it may be necessary to use composite grafts to overcome mucosal deficit.

It must be admitted that complete elimination of alar notching may not be possible.

Lobular Deformities

Imperfections of the tip are common after primary rhinoplasty and range from simple lack of definition to defacement. Although sometimes resulting from the limitations imposed by the quality of the patient's skin, anatomy, and a history of previous nasal trauma, many represent errors of omission or commission or are caused by scar contracture intranasally.

The external approach has been a boon to the performance of secondary rhinoplasty because the surgeon can clearly see the cause and extent of the deformity and immediately determine the effectiveness of the corrective measures used. We cannot recommend it too highly.

An integral part of most secondary lobular deformities is a supratip accumulation of hypertrophic scar tissue that spills over onto the caudal ends of the upper lateral cartilages. It must be detached from the undersurface of the skin; otherwise, satisfactory skin drapeage becomes almost impossible.

We address the problem by keeping the plane of dissection immediately subdermal when undermining the overlying skin so that the scarred mass remains attached to the skeletal structures and becomes easier to remove later. The technique reestablishes the pliability of the overlying skin.

After the cartilages have been exposed, they are mobilized and restored to their usual location; if necessary, an attempt is made to correct unwelcome curves, and properly shaped implants of crushed cartilage are used to fill any remaining depressions or dehiscences or to cover any sharp edges.

At the end of remodeling, the septal dorsum should be made level with the apexes of the nostrils and the tip bandaged in that position.

Some lobules are so badly mangled that they defy the efforts of even the most expert and intrepid surgeons to achieve even modest improvement. Their repair is best left in the hands of those experts who are willing to accept the challenge.

Vestibular Scarring

Scarring of the vestibule is due to lining deficit caused by too generous excision of vestibular skin and the contiguous mucous membrane or by poor placement or closure of incisions. In rare cases, Z-plasty or other types of flap rotation may be successful; however, it is usually necessary to excise the scars and fill the deficit with composite or full-thickness skin grafts.

Septal Adhesions

Septal adhesions sometimes seem to arise by spontaneous generation, but they are probably due to small, overlooked lacerations of the mucosa of the septum or apposing turbinates; they usually respond favorably to lysis on one or more occasions. More difficult to resolve are those that occur between the septum and the undersurface of the nasal pyramid; some of these have thwarted our best efforts up to and including total excision followed by rotation of flaps of septal mucosa.

We have encountered septal adhesions that have formed several months after rhinoplasty, so it behooves surgeons to do intranasal examinations after operation.

Nasal Valve Collapse

The place where the caudal ends of the upper lateral cartilages meet the septal dorsum has been termed the "nasal valves." They do not impede airflow during quiet respiration, but they will close down during forceful inspiration or when the angles are stiffened or lessened secondary to rhinoplasty. In most cases, the problem can be traced to septal deviation, be it ever so slight, in the valve area. Straightening the septum clears up the problem in such instances. However, valvular collapse can occur when too much cartilage is excised from the lateral crura, when scar tissue from improperly placed limen vestibula incisions lessen the upper lateral cartilage-septal angle and stiffen the adjacent limen, and when the upper lateral cartilages lack enough rigidity to cope with the negative pressure generated during normal respiration.

Cartilage battens obtained from the nasal septum or the ear may be used to correct collapse due to excessive removal of lateral crura and, sometimes, when the upper lateral cartilages are weakened or deficient; these battens usually cause some fullness in the areas in which they are used, but most patients feel this is preferable to the alternative.

Composite grafts are used when there is need for lining in addition to skeletal replacement.

The success of valve repair is often very tenuous, so a simultaneous effort should be made to keep the negative pressure required for inspiratory comfort to a minimum. This may require submucous resection of the inferior turbinate or, as has been mentioned, septal straightening; of course, any concurrent nasal allergy should be treated.

18   Chin Augmentation

Many of the patients who seek rhinoplasty do not realize that the relationship of the nose to the chin and the forehead cannot be ignored when attempting to achieve profile balance. Thus, the surgeon is often obliged to educate and advise patients of their need for chin augmentation or, more rarely, for chin reduction.

The element of surprise on the part of the patient can be reduced and acceptance facilitated by sending them informational material to read in advance of the initial consultation. Having photographs to depict their problem is, also, helpful.

We find that correction of a receding chin is necessary at the time of rhinoplasty in from 15 to 20 percent of the cases in order to create a harmonious profile.

Two types of chin recession encountered are microgenia and micrognathia. In microgenia, the chin eminence is diminished, but the mandible is satisfactory; if slight malocclusion is present, it is not functionally disturbing. Correction of microgenia with modern allographs is fairly simple for both the surgeon and the patient in contrast to bygone days when hip grafts were widely used; fortunately, the results of allographs are remarkably good. Micrognathia, on the other hand, features occlusal and mandibular disturbances and should be referred to appropriate professionals for correction.

In the past, we have used bone, autogenous and homogenous cartilage, acrylic, solid silicone, and silicone sponge and have encountered problems with all of them. For the past several years, we have used gel-filled silicone chin implants (manufactured by the McGhan Medical Corporation of Santa Barbara, California) and have never had any troubles with them. They are available in six different sizes, and the soft gel makes them flexible enough to be inserted through a small incision and allows them to conform to the bony mentum.

Likewise, for many years we used the intraoral approach for augmentation. However, about 10 years ago, we switched to the external approach, not because we were experiencing postoperative infections, but to enhance patient comfort during eating; we have never regretted the decision to change and have found that the submental incision becomes virtually imperceptible in a short time, provided it is properly located and sutured.

As is the case with the nose, the amount of correction necessary is determined in advance by photographic analysis. However, a rapid, rough estimate may be made by dropping a vertical line from the vermilion border of the lower lip when a well-posed profile view is available; ideally, the profile of the chin should touch that line, but very satisfying improvement can be achieved for many patients, even if it falls somewhat short of the mark.

When combined with rhinoplasty, chin augmentation should always be completed first, because it may alter one's plan for correcting the nose; for example, a receding chin may lead one to believe that a major correction of the nose is indicated, but the nasal change need not be so drastic after the projection of the chin has been increased.

TECHNIQUE

1. The chin is marked as indicated in Figure 113a. Essentially, three vertical and three horizontal lines are constructed. The middle vertical line corresponds to the space between the central incisor teeth; the location of the lateral lines are determined by the space between the lateral incisors and the canines. The first horizontal line lies at the level of the gingival sulcus, the second along the margin of the mandible, and the third is plotted halfway between the other two. These markings define where the implant will be centered.

2. The mental and immediate submental areas are infiltrated with 2% lidocaine containing 1:100,000 epinephrine.

3. Ten minutes later, an incision about 2 cm long is made in the submental crease with an electric scalpel (Shaw); this cut extends through the dermis only (Fig. 113b).

4. The upper margin of the wound is retracted

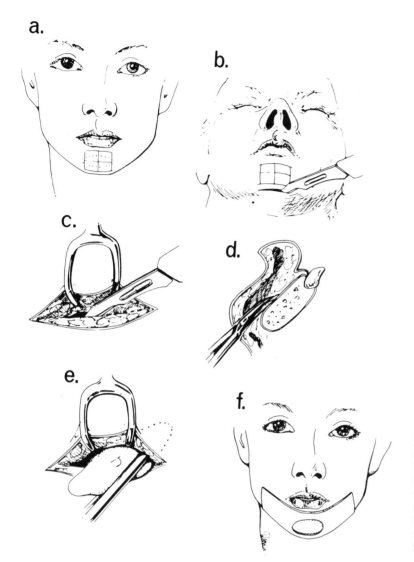

Figure 113. a: Markings used when planning chin augmentation. b: Incision is made through skin only. c: Incision is continued down to the periosteum while the upper edge of the wound is retracted cephalically. d: Soft tissues are cut away from the periosteum. e: Gel-filled silicone implant is inserted into pocket. f: Dressing is applied for 3 days.

cephalically with a small rake retractor, and the subcutaneous fat is incised down to, but not through, the mental periosteum (Fig. 113c).

5. The tissues overlying the chin are elevated by cutting them from the periosteum with an iris scissors to create a pocket (Fig. 113d) bounded by the upper and lower horizontal and the lateral vertical lines previously plotted on the skin. Care is taken during the dissection not to puncture the gingivolabial sulcus and not to injure the mental nerves that exit through foramina lying below the first permolar teeth. Aside from the entrance, the tissues attached to the mandibular margin should not be disturbed.

6. Any bleeding vessels are cauterized.

7. An appropriately sized sterile implant that has been soaked in Gentamicin solution is introduced with a dressing forceps (Fig. 113e), and a flattened instrument is passed above and below its entire length to be certain that the implant was not bent on itself during introduction. Additionally, one must be sure that the blue dot that marks the center of the implant is properly aligned.

8. Two sutures of 4–0 chromic catgut with inverted knots are inserted to coapt the subdermal tissues.

9. The skin is closed with several mattress sutures of 4–0 polypropylene.

10. An antibiotic ointment is applied to the sutured incision before covering it with a small piece of Telfa.

11. A dressing of Microform tape with a cutout section to immobilize the implant for 3 days is applied (Fig. 113f). When the tape is removed, the sutures are also removed; then, the wound is supported with Steri-Strips for 4 additional days.

19 Case Discussions

We have not used before and after photographs of patients in the text to illustrate the effectiveness of specific technical steps because we firmly believe that individual adjustments are best viewed and evaluated within the context of the total correction. Thus, this chapter is devoted to a discussion of a number of cases of varying degrees of complexity. They were chosen to illustrate the application of many of the principles that we discussed. We will relate what our main surgical aims were before operation and describe how we tried to solve the problems encountered.

It is interesting to note that we failed to achieve a score of 100 in any of these cases; the improvement varied from 20 to 30 percent in our opinion. The reader might find it an interesting exercise to grade the patients noses before and after operation to determine how effective the efforts were and where we failed; we use the Rhinoplasty Scale depicted in Figure 112 to grade noses before and after operation. Essentially, 1 or 2 points are subtracted for each defect, and the total is subtracted from 100.

Incidentally, all postoperative photographs were taken at least 1 year after surgery unless otherwise noted.

FIGURE 114

Note that the postoperative views were converted to black and white from Kodachrome transparencies taken in January 1985.

Etiology: congenital
Surgical approach: external
Surgical aims: Rotate and increase projection of tip, narrow lobule, level hump

Surgical Problems and Their Solution

1. Hump: bone leveled with rasp, cartilage with scissors
2. Septum: Killian procedure to facilitate later narrowing of pyramid
3. Nasal base
   a. The alar cartilages were separated from each other by cutting the intracrural ligaments, and the scroll of each lateral crus was removed intramucosally, leaving approximately 5 mm of each crus behind
   b. Each alar cartilage was divided intramucosally at the angle, and the vestibular skin was dissected from the medial ends of the lateral crura for a distance of 5 to 7 mm
   c. The upper ends of the medial crura were narrowed by 50 per cent; the remaining cartilage was coapted with a mattress suture through the adjacent vestibular skin
   d. A small triangle of cartilage was excised intramucosally from the lateral ends of the lateral crura to permit entad rotation of those structures
   e. The medial ends of the lateral crura that overlapped the upper ends of the medial crura were trimmed so that they abutted each other and the medial crura; the underlying vestibular skin was coapted with mattress sutures
4. Nasal shortening: accomplished by shortening the medial ends of the lateral crura after the medial crura had been rotated until they abutted the caudal end of the nasal septum; no septal cartilage was excised

Figure 114.

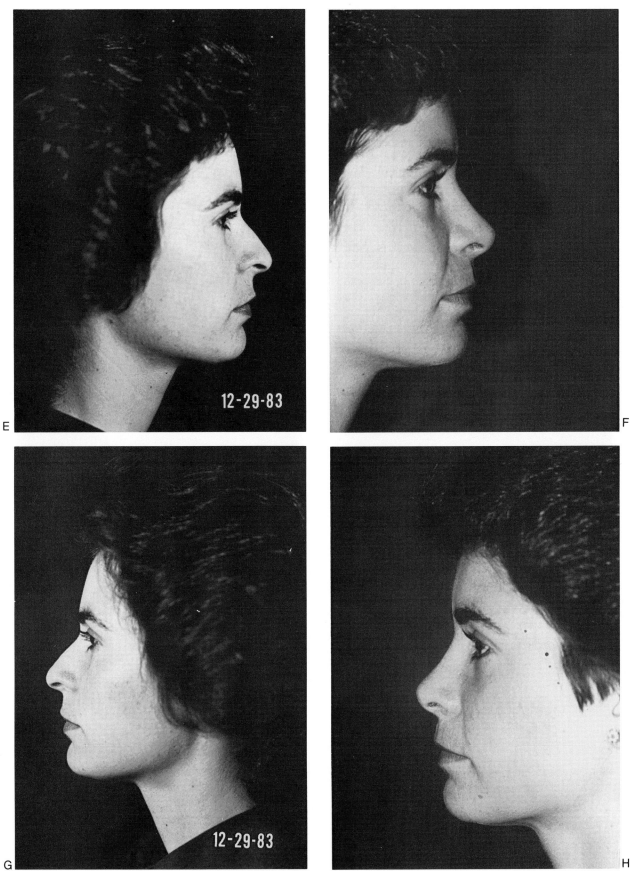

Figure 114.

FIGURE 115

Note that the postoperative views were converted to black and white from Kodachrome transparencies taken in June 1982.

Etiology: congenital
Surgical approach: external
Surgical aim: to reduce tip projection without shortening the nose; plan was to shorten both legs of the nasal base tripod

Surgical Problems and Their Solution

1. Thin, aging skin: dissection kept close to skeleton
2. Large hump: leveled with Rubin chisel, scalpel, and scissors
3. Narrowing: submucous resection of septum beneath the bony pyramid was necessary
4. Reduction of excessive tip projection:
   a. Excision of cartilage from inferior septal angle to shorten short leg of the nasal base tripod
   b. Lowering projection of the septal dorsum
   c. Excision of cartilage segments from lateral ends of the lateral crura to shorten long legs of the tripod
5. Lobule refinement: intact rim technique used
6. Prevention of nasal base rotation; mobilization of scroll area but little excision

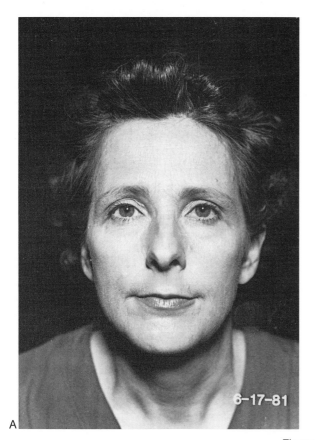 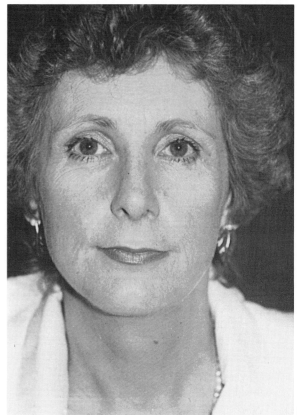

A   B

Figure 115.

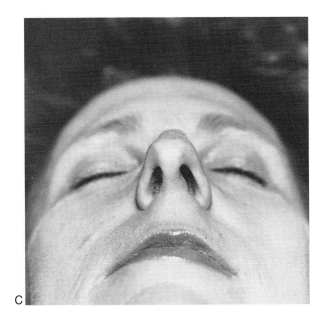

C

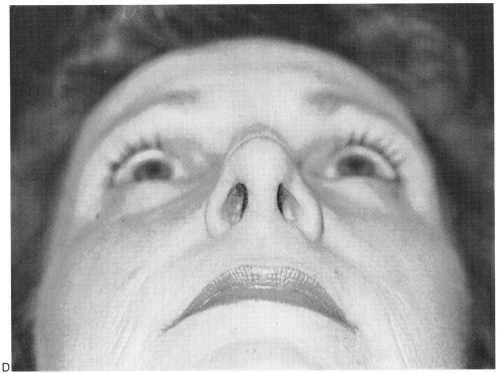

D

Figure 115.

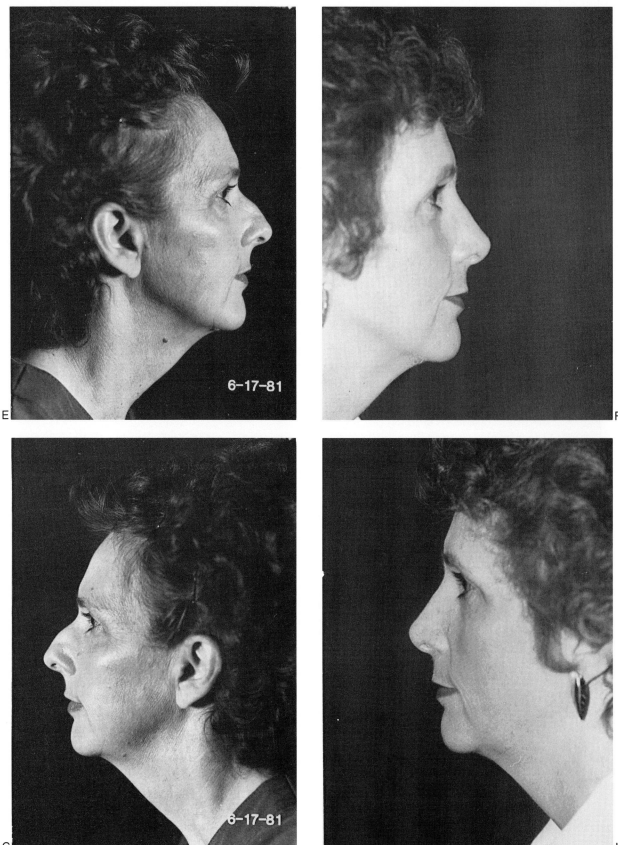

Figure 115.

FIGURE 116

Note that the postoperative views were converted to black and white from Kodachrome transparencies taken in March 1982.

Etiology: congenital
Surgical approach: external
Surgical aims: to decrease tip projection markedly; to rotate and correct the asymmetry of the lobule; to correct the wideness of the base of the columella and the pseudo-webbing of the nasolabial angle; to straighten the cartilagenous dorsum

Surgical Problems and Solutions

1. Hump: projection of cartilagenous dorsum reduced
2. Septum
   a. Killian submucous resection of posterior compartment
   b. Swinging-door procedure performed to correct dislocation of the caudal section of the septal cartilage and to straighten the cartilagenous dorsum
   c. Lipping of the nasal spine corrected
   d. Cartilage was excised from the inferior septal angle to allow the feet of the medial crura to subside in the direction of the premaxillae
3. Nasal base
   a. The alar cartilages were incised intramucosally at their angles
   b. A wedge of cartilage was excised at each angle to triangulate the lobule; more cartilage was excised on the right side to correct asymmetry
   c. The scrolls of the lateral crura were excised
   d. A segment of cartilage was excised from each lateral crus just lateral to their bodies to shorten the longer legs of the tripod to permit lobular rotation and to permit the tripod to descend toward the facial plane
   e. Soft tissue was excised from beneath the feet of the medial crura, and the flaring lower ends of those structures were transected so they could be moved medially to narrow the base of the columella
   f. An intracrural shoring strut of septal cartilage was introduced to limit tip subsidence
   g. Wedge resections from the nostril floors were performed to overcome the widening of the alae that occurred secondary to the marked reduction of tip projection

NOTE: Simultaneous chin augmentation was not advised pending determination of the effect of tip recession on the profile; chin projection seemed acceptable after rhinoplasty.

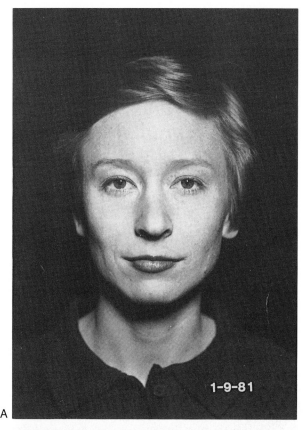

1-9-81

A

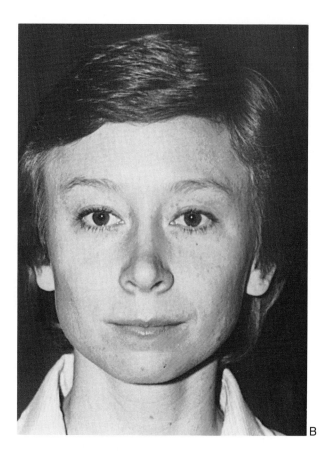

B

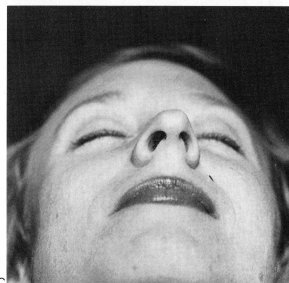

C

Figure 116.

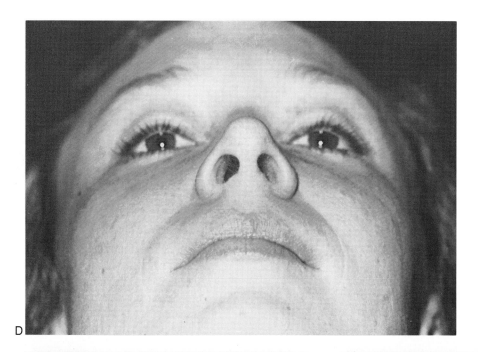

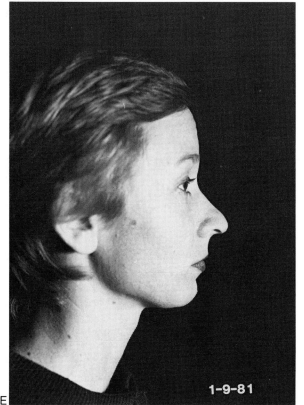

1-9-81

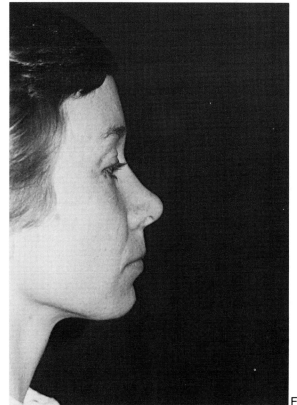

Figure 116.

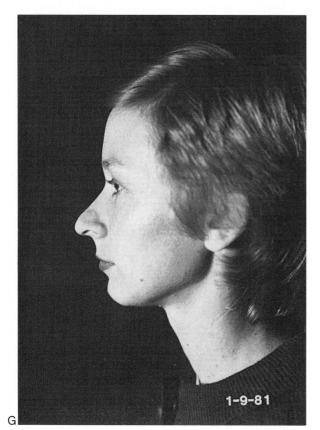
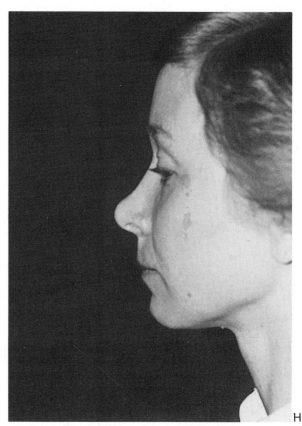

1-9-81

G   H

Figure 116.

FIGURE 117

Note that the postoperative views were converted to black and white from Kodachrome transparencies taken in February 1983.

Etiology: congenital
Surgical approach: external
Surgical aims: To narrow, rotate, and increase projection of the lobule; to correct flaring of the feet of the medial crura and the hanging columella; to level the nasal hump

Surgical Problems and Solutions

1. Nasal septum: Killian submucous resection beneath the hump; no shortening of the caudal lend of the septum
2. Nasal hump: leveled intramucosally with a rasp and scalpel blade after tip was rotated and its projection set
3. Pyramid narrowing
   a. Medial and lateral osteotomies were performed
   b. "Returning" of the upper lateral cartilages was corrected to eliminate widening of the lateral supratip area
4. Nasal base:
   a. The alar cartilages were incised intramucosally at their angles
   b. The caudal ends of the lateral crura were denuded of vestibular skin for a distance of 5 to 7 mm; the skin was also dissected away from the upper 3 mm of the medial crura; this maneuver caused the cartilages to straighten
   c. The width of the upper ends of the medial crura was reduced by 50 percent
   d. The scrolls of the lateral crura abutting the caudal ends of the upper lateral crura were excised
   e. Triangular segments of cartilage, base directed cephalically, were excised from each lateral crus just lateral to its body to permit rotation of that structure
   f. The medial crura were transected just above the flaring of their feet so that part of the columella could be narrowed by suturing

g. Cartilage was excised from the caudal borders of the medial crura to correct the hanging columella

h. An intracrural shoring strut of autogenous cartilage was introduced to maintain tip projection

i. The medial ends of the lateral crura were appropriately trimmed to shorten them and to establish the proper relationship with each other and with the medial crura

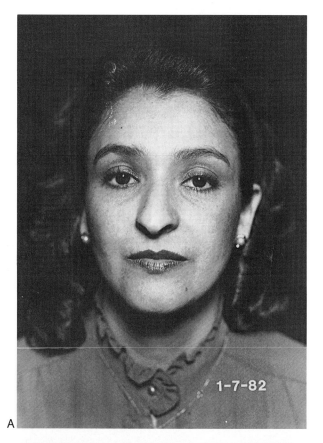

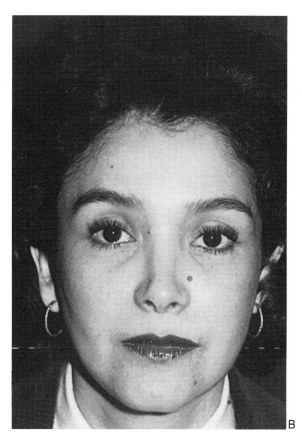

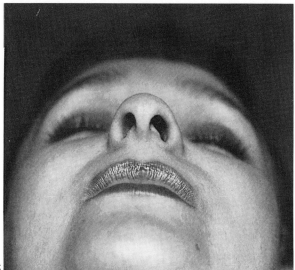

Figure 117.

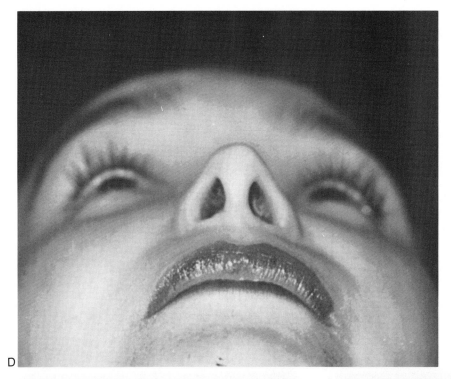

D

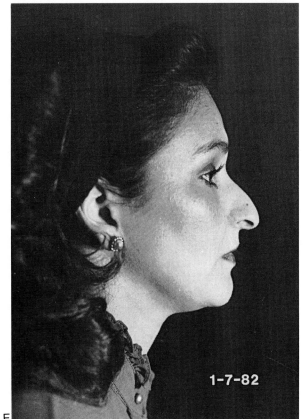

E

1-7-82

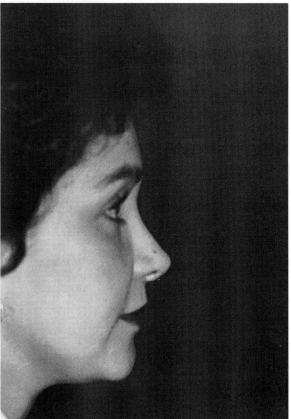

F

Figure 117.

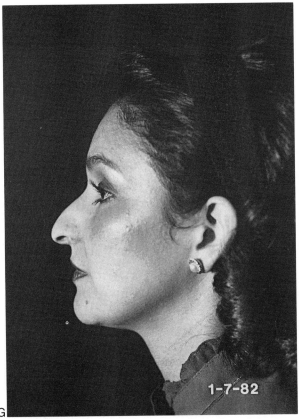

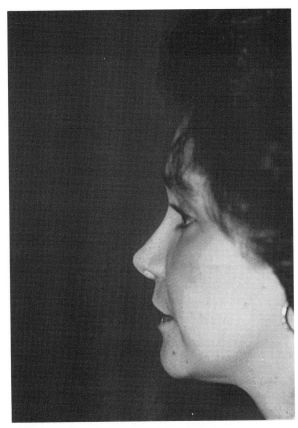

1-7-82

G   H

Figure 117.

FIGURE 118

Note that the preoperative views were taken in June 1974. Postoperative views were converted to black and white from Kodachrome transparencies taken in May 1977.

Etiology: congenital
Surgical approach: endonasal
Surgical aims: to narrow and shorten the nose, refine the lobule and reduce the thickness of the subcutaneous tissue

Surgical Problems and Solutions

1. Skin: excessive subcutaneous tissues were dissected from the undersurface of the skin of the lower half, and the undersurface of the subdermis in the supratip area was crosshatched with a scalpel blade
2. Hump: leveled with a rasp
3. Narrowing
   a. Widened dorsal edge of septal cartilage narrowed
   b. Submucous resection beneath pyramid; dorsal buttress preserved
   c. Double osteotomies
   d. Excision of segments of nasal bones remaining attached to frontal spine after pyramid mobilization
   e. Mucosa dissected away from undersurface of medial ends of upper lateral cartilages for a distance of 3 mm
   f. "Returning" of upper lateral cartilages excised
4. Nasal base
   a. Alar cartilages divided intramucosally at their angles
   b. Lateral crural scrolls excised bilaterally
   c. Vestibular skin dissected away from the medial ends of the lateral crura for distance of 5 to 7 mm; this caused medial ends to straighten
   d. Soft tissue was excised from between the feet of the medial crura to narrow the base of the columella
   e. An intracrural strut of septal cartilage was inserted
   f. The cut ends of the medial crura were sewn together

g. Medial ends of the lateral crura were trimmed to abut each other and the medial crura

5. Nasal shortening: accomplished by scroll excision, dividing alae at angles, and excising cartilage from the medial ends of the lateral crura and by excising a triangular segment of cartilages, base directed cephalically, from the lateral ends of the lateral crura

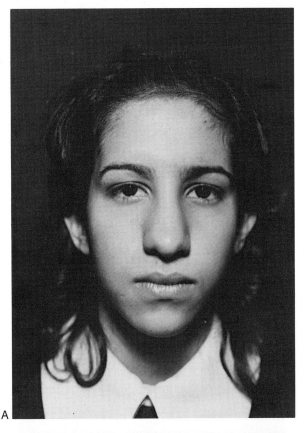
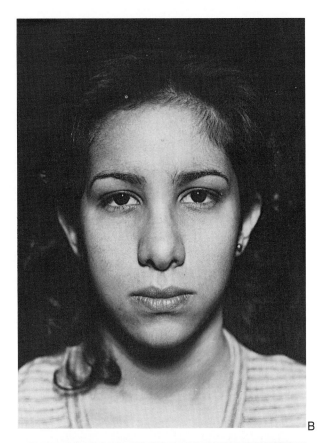
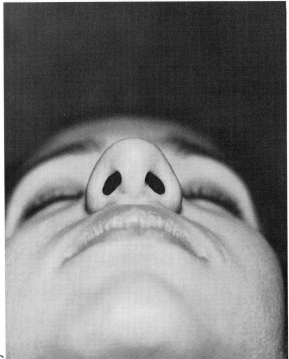
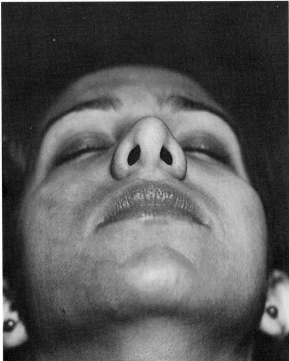

Figure 118.

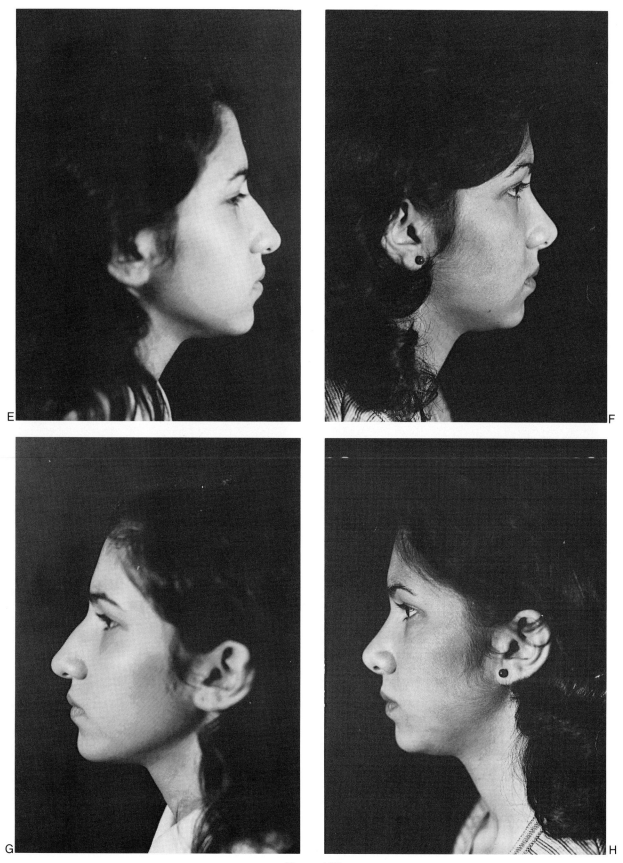

Figure 118.

FIGURE 119

Note that the preoperative photos were taken April 1979.

Etiology: congenital
Surgical approach: external
Surgical aim: to narrow pyramid and tip and correct saddle deformity

Surgical Problems and Corrections

1. Deviated septum: Killian submucous resection
2. Narrowing pyramid
   a. Medial and lateral osteotomies
   b. Mucosa dissected away from undersurface of medial ends of upper lateral cartilages for a distance of about 3 mm
   c. Two layers of ear cartilage placed along entire length of the nasal dorsum

3. Nasal base
   a. Alar cartilages divided intramucosally at their angles
   b. Small amount of scrolls excised from lateral crura
   c. Vestibular skin dissected away from the medial ends of the lateral crura for a distance of about 7 mm
   d. Intracrural strut of septal cartilage inserted to improve tip projection
   e. Cut ends of medial crura narrowed and sewn together
   f. Button of morselized cartilage placed above sewn ends of medial crura to increase their length
   g. Medial ends of lateral crura trimmed and leaned against lengthened upper ends of medial crura
   h. Wedge resections from nostril sills to narrow alae
   i. Mild tip rotation accomplished transecting alae and trimming medial ends of lateral crura

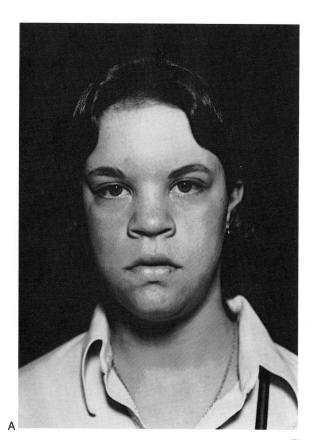

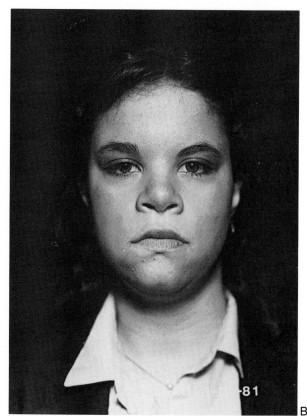

A   B

Figure 119.

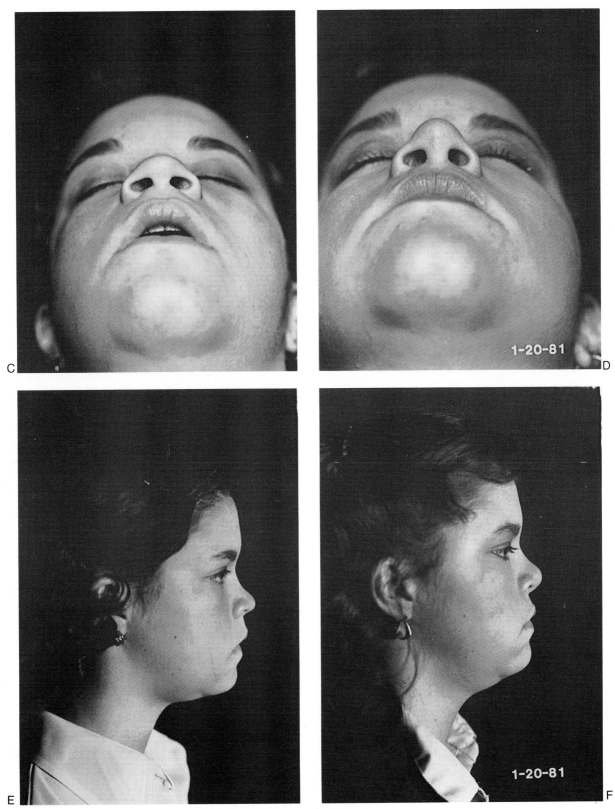

Figure 119.

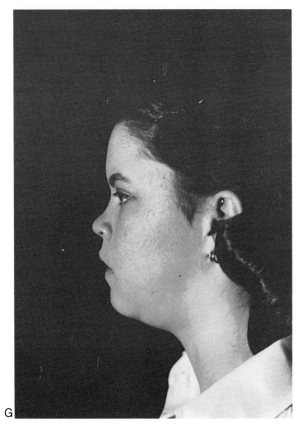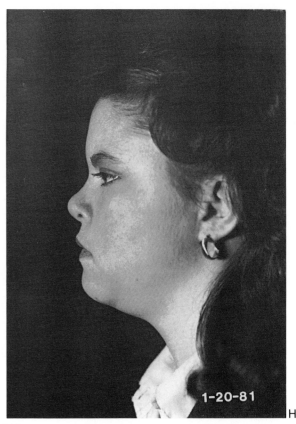

Figure 119.

FIGURE 120

Note that the postoperative photos were converted to black and white from Kodachrome transparencies taken in November 1984.

Etiology: congenital
Surgical approach: external
Surgical aims: narrow nose, improve projection of the nasal dorsum and nasal tip, improve appearance of base

Surgical Problems and Solutions

1. Septum: Killian submucous resection performed beneath pyramid
2. Narrowing: Intramucosally after medial and lateral osteotomies; the medial borders of the upper lateral cartilages were denuded of mucosa for a distance of 3 mm
3. Saddling: Three layers of morselized autogenous and bank cartilage were placed along the entire length of the nasal dorsum
4. Nasal base
   a. Excessive supratip soft tissues were removed and the undersurface of the dermis was crosshatched
   b. The alar cartilages were incised intramucosally at their angles
   c. The vestibular skin was dissected from the undersurface of the medial ends of the lateral crura for a distance of 5 to 7 mm
   d. Three layers of morselized cartilage were implanted over the premaxillae after the adjacent soft tissues were elevated from the surrounding bones
   e. A shoring strut of septal cartilage was sewn between the medial crura; it extended from the premaxillary implants to the cut ends of the medial crura
   f. The medial crura were lengthened by laying three layers of cartilage above their upper ends
   g. The denuded medial ends of the lateral crura were converted to projectors of the tip by leaning them against the lengthened medial crura; they were trimmed appropriately
   h. Wedges of tissue were excised from the nostril margins to narrow the alae

NOTE: This patient rejected the recommendation for chin augmentation.

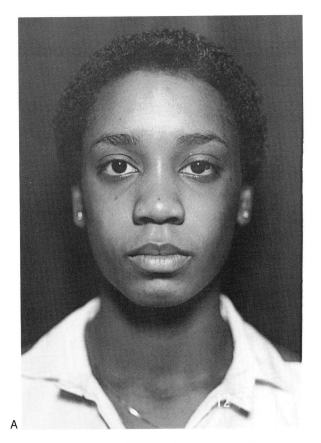

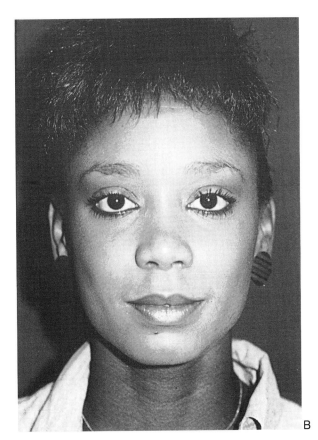

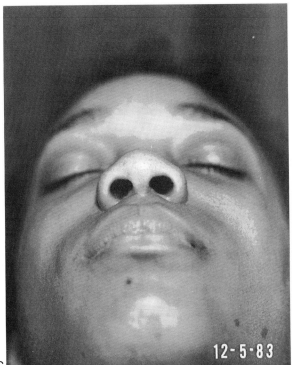

Figure 120.

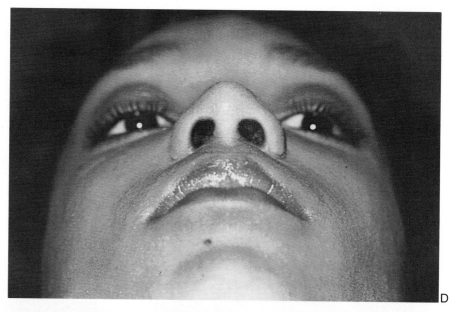

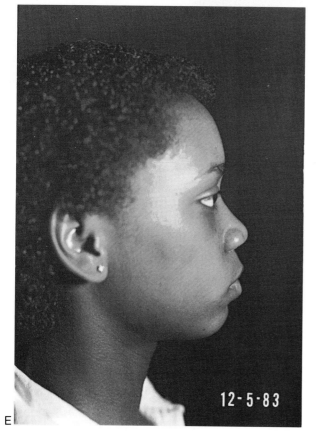

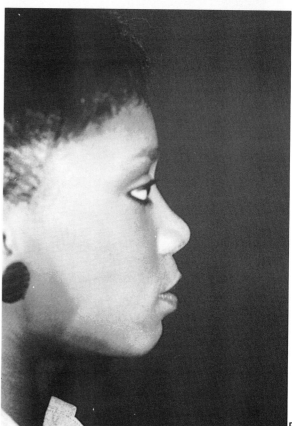

Figure 120.

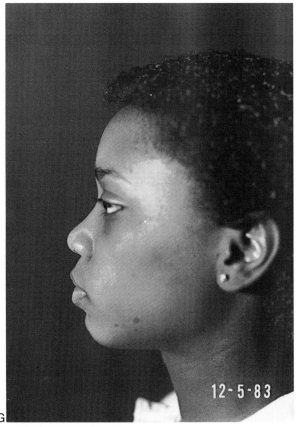

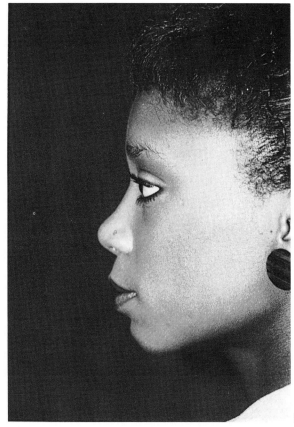

Figure 120.

FIGURE 121

Note that the postoperative photos were converted to black and white from Kodachrome transparencies taken in August 1982.

Etiology: congenital cleft lip nose; lip previously repaired
Surgical approach: external
Surgical aims: to narrow nasal pyramid and lobule; to increase lobular projection with minimal shortening of the dorsum; to correct lobular and nostril asymmetry and to correct a deviated and dislocated nasal septum

Surgical Problems and Solutions

1. Hump: minor leveling of the dorsum with a rasp and scalpel
2. Nasal septum
   a. Killian submucous resection of posterior segment
   b. Swinging-door septoplasty of caudal segment
   c. Lipping of the nasal spine corrected
3. Narrowing: after medial and double lateral osteotomies
4. Nasal base

a. Small amount of scrolls excised from the lateral crura bilaterally
b. The alar cartilages were separated by cutting all of the intracrural ligaments
c. Triangular wedges of cartilage were excised from the angles of both alar cartilages; a large wedge was excised from the normal side
d. The premaxilla was exposed via the separated medial crura and the soft tissues were elevated from the surrounding bone
e. The skin of the upper lip was undermined
f. Three layers of morselized cartilage were placed on the premaxilla beneath the base of the medial crura
g. An intracrural strut of septal cartilage was sewn in place, and the columella base was narrowed
h. A morselized layer of thin septal cartilage was cut to pattern and implanted over the alar dome on the cleft side to equalize projection
i. The alar base on the cleft side was moved medially

NOTE: The scar of the lip was subsequently revised.

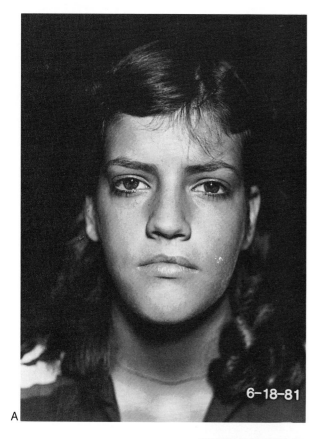

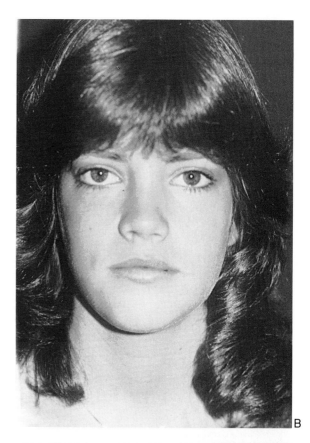

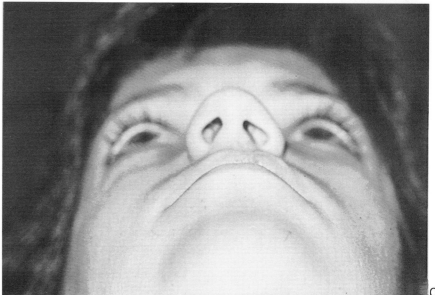

Figure 121.

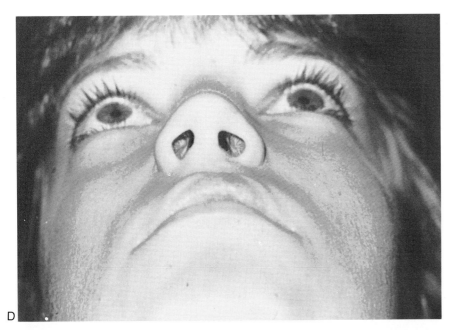

D

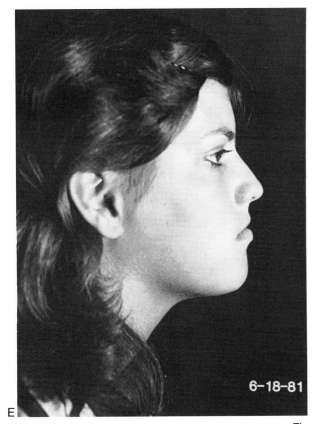

E

6-18-81

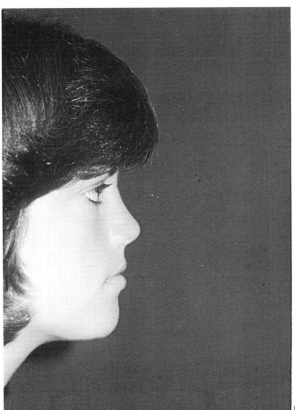

F

Figure 121.

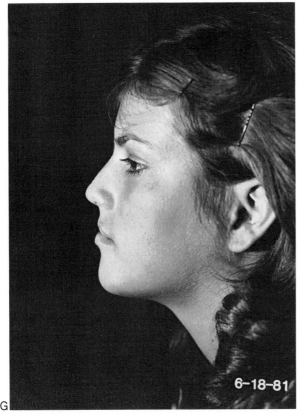

6-18-81

G

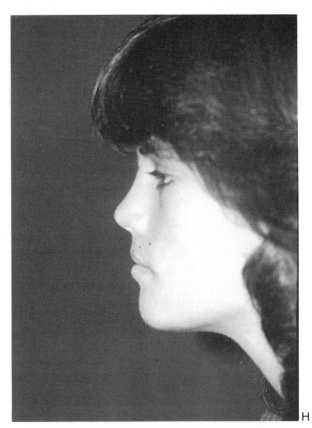

H

Figure 121.

FIGURE 122

Note that the preoperative photographs were taken November 1979, and the postoperative photographs were taken September 1981.

Etiology: congenital; classic maxillofacial triad of Goldman

Surgical problems: Nasal hump with shallow nasofrontal angle, curvature of cartilagenous dorsum to left, insufficient tip projection, nasal dorsum slightly elongated, nasolabial angle retracted, insufficient chin projection

Approach: nose—endonasal; chin—intraoral

Corrective Procedures

1. Hump, shallow nasofrontal angle
   a. Avulsion of procerus muscle with narrow Lempert rongeur
   b. Bony hump removed and nasofrontal angle deepened simultaneously with Rubin osteotome driven as close as possible to the nasofrontal suture line

2. Curvature of nasal dorsum
   a. Killian submucous resection, plus swinging-door procedure to correct caudal septum
   b. Nasal spine straightened by cutting it on bias
   c. Caudal segment splinted for 7 days
   d. Projection of upper lateral cartilages equalized; "returning" of caudal ends corrected

3. Nasal base
   a. Lobule refined and rotated with intact rim technique after cartilage-splitting incisions; 5 mm of each lateral crus left behind
   b. Nasolabial angle projection improved by nasal base rotation
   c. Intracrural shoring strut of septal cartilage used to ensure postoperative maintenance of tip projection and to help improve nasolabial angle retraction

4. Shortening the nose
   a. Accomplished by nasal base rotation; there was no shortening of the caudal end of the septum

5. Improved chin projection

a. Solid silicone implant used via intraoral approach

Grade of Nose

Preoperative: 71.
Postoperative: 98.

Criticism

The preoperative profile views obviously do not meet the standards of good rhinoplasty photography.

Some nostril asymmetry remains, and the desirable supratip break was not achieved.

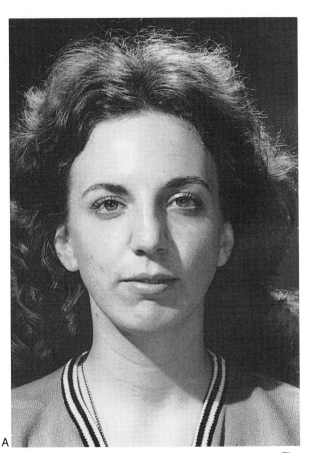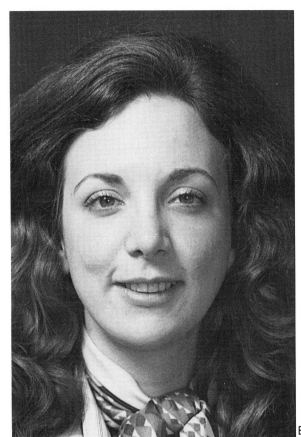

Figure 122.

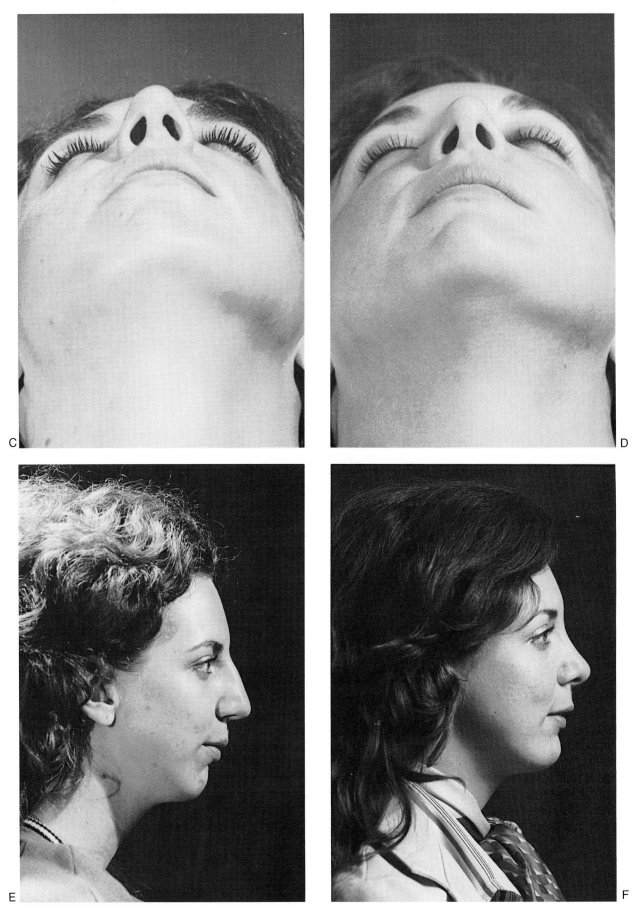

C

D

E

F

Figure 122.

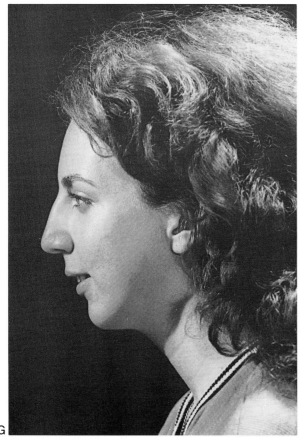
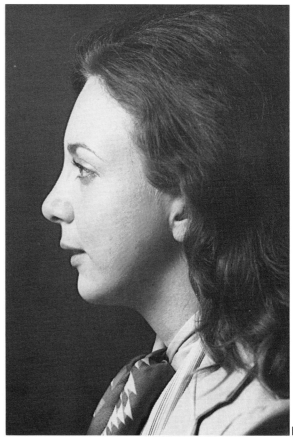

G   H

Figure 122.

FIGURE 123

Etiology: congenital and ethnic (Mayan)
Surgical approach: external
Surgical aims: to rotate and increase the projection of the tip, narrow the lobule and reduce the width of the alae, reduce the thickness of the soft tissue in the tip and supratip area, correct a fractured nasal septum, increase chin projection

Surgical Problems and Their Solutions

1. Thinning tip and supratip soft tissues
   a. Dissection from the overlying skin
   b. Crosshatching the undersurface of the dermis to effect increased skin pliability
2. Reduction of the width of the lobule
   a. The alar cartilages were divided intramucosally at their angles
   b. Small strips of cartilage were removed from the scroll areas
   c. The medial ends of the lateral crura were denuded of vestibular skin for a distance of about 5 mm
   d. The caudal ends of the upper lateral cartilages were shortened
3. Tip rotation and increased projection
   a. A septal cartilage strut was inserted into the columella; it extended from just above the premaxillae to the apexes of the nostrils
   b. The upper ends of the medial crura were lengthened with an onlay graft of cartilage
   c. The medial ends of the lateral crura, now straighter because they had previously been denuded of vestibular skin, were leaned against the elongated medial crura to increase their effectiveness as projectors of the tip
4. The fractured nasal septum was corrected by means of a classic Killian submucous resection
5. Hump removal was accomplished with a Rubin osteotome, a rasp, and scissors
6. Reduction of alae width was accomplished by wedge resections from the nostrils
7. Chin projection was increased with a no. 2 gel-filled implant (McGhan) inserted through a submental incision

Figure 123.

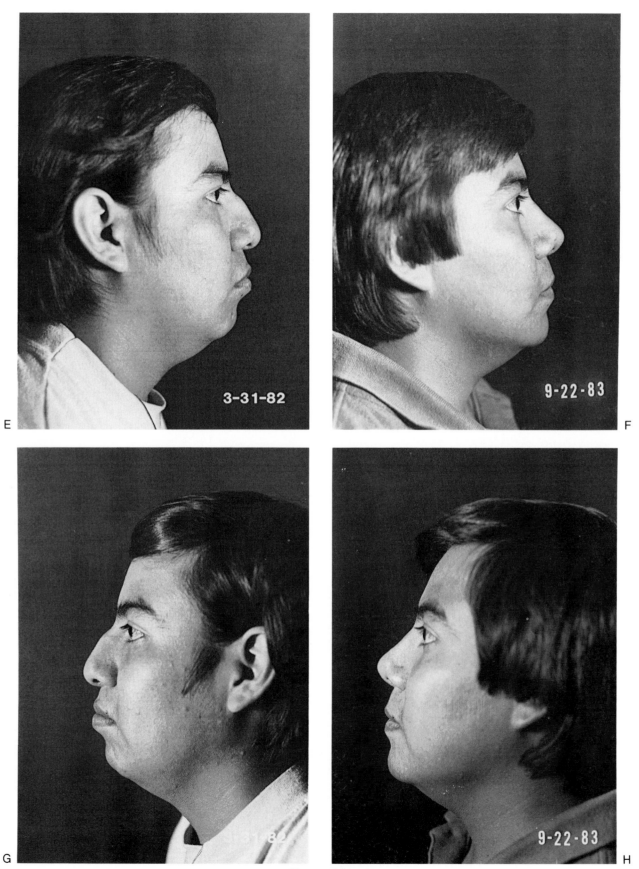

Figure 123.

FIGURE 124

Etiology: traumatic during childhood
Surgical approach: external
Surgical aims: to straighten nose; correct supratip
saddling; reduce tip projection, ro-
tate it, and reduce its width

Surgical Problems and Their Solutions

1. Bony hump
   a. Leveled with a rasp
   b. Dorsal implants consisting of two
      layers of morselized autogenous
      septal cartilage
2. Nasal septum
   a. Killian submucous resection of pos-
      terior segment
   b. Swinging-door septoplasty of cau-
      dal end
   c. Nasal spine straightened by cutting
      it on bias

d. The medial 3 mm of the left upper
   lateral cartilage was denuded of mucosa
3. Mobilization of lateral walls of the bony
   pyramid: by medial and lateral osteotomies
4. Nasal base:
   a. A small amount of cartilage was
      excised from the lateral crural
      scrolls
   b. Both alar cartilages were cut intra-
      mucosally at their angles and the
      underlying mucosa was dissected
      free from the medial 3 to 5 mm of
      each lateral crus
   c. A small triangle of cartilage, base
      directed upward, was removed from
      each lateral crus just lateral to its
      body
   d. The ends of the lateral crura that
      were in excess after rotation were
      excised and trimmed appropriately
      so they abutted the medial crura
      and each other

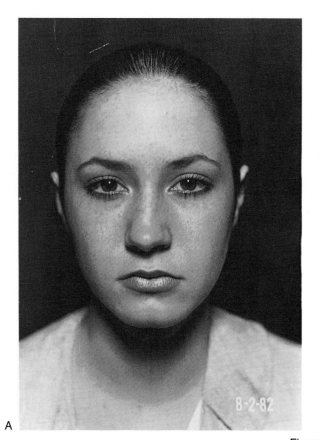 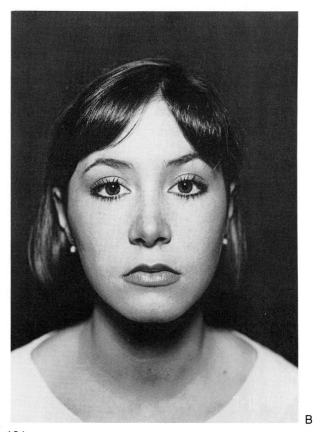

A   B

Figure 124.

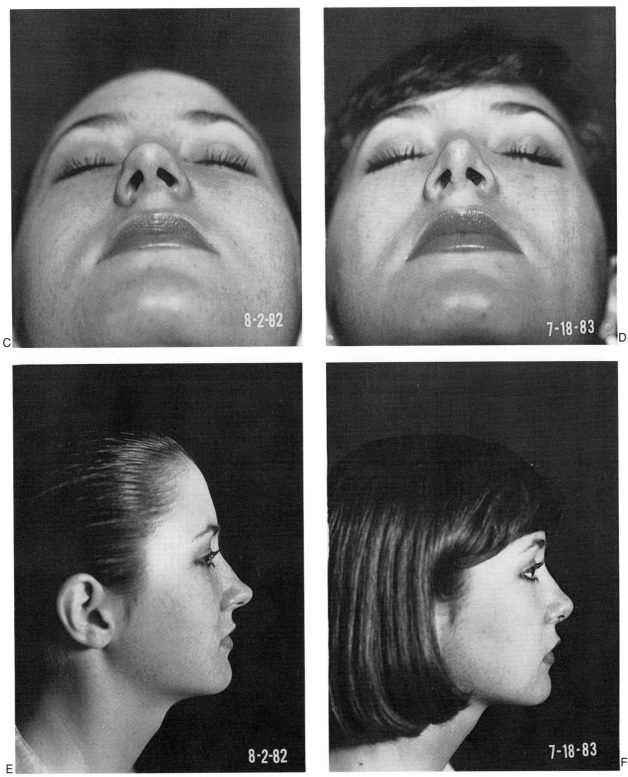

Figure 124.

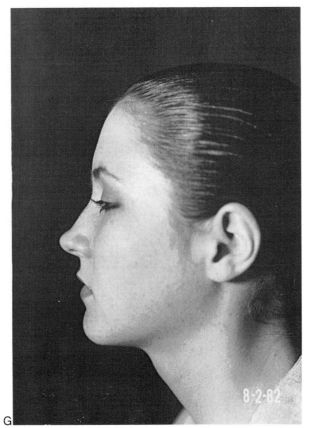
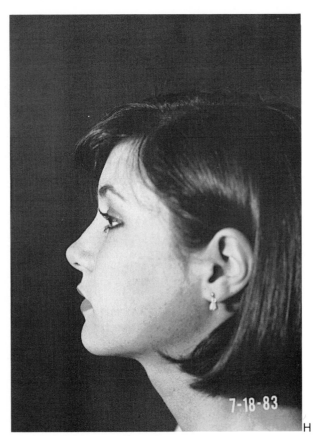

Figure 124.

FIGURE 125

Note that all views were converted to black and white from Kodachrome transparencies. Preoperative views were taken January 1980, and postoperative views were taken May 1981.

Etiology: post-traumatic
Surgical approach: external
Surgical aims: to straighten nose and recontour
dorsum

Surgical Problems and Their Solution

1. Hump: Rasped
2. Saddling: Three layers of morselized and crushed cartilage implanted along the entire dorsum
3. Deviation of bony and cartilagenous dorsum
   a. Killian submucous resection and swinging-door procedure
   b. Nasal spine straightened
   c. Equalization of projection of upper lateral cartilages
   d. Caudal ends of upper lateral cartilages shortened
4. Nasal base
   a. Knuckling of right dome: cartilage projection caused by old fracture leveled by excision
   b. Widened lobule: scrolls of lateral crura excised; rim of cartilage around nostrils preserved
   c. Decreased tip projection: corrected by straightening caudal septum by morselization and shifting it to midline and by use of an intracrural shoring strut of cartilage
   d. Retracted columella: corrected by shoring strut
   e. Widened alae: corrected by wedge resections
5. Excessive nasal length: lateral crura rotated by excision of triangular segment from their lateral ends

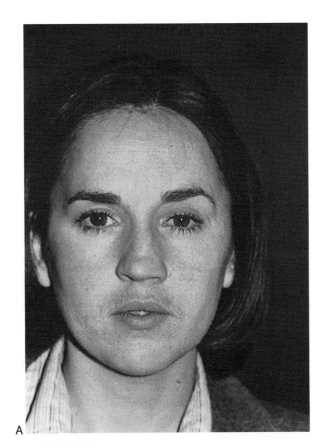

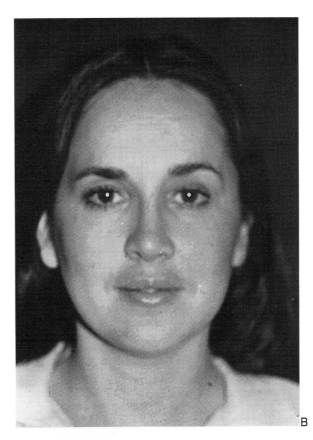

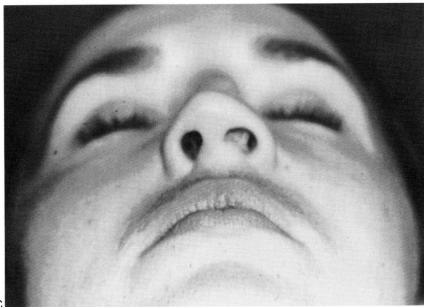

Figure 125.

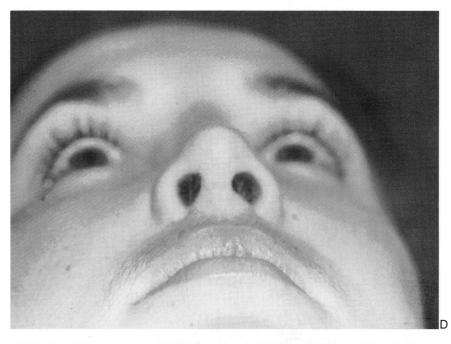

D

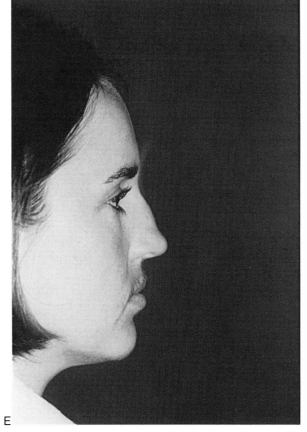

E

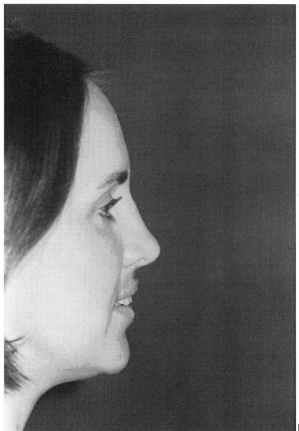

F

Figure 125.

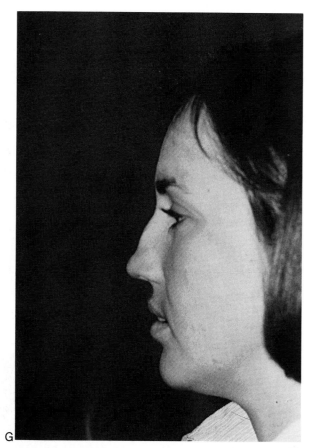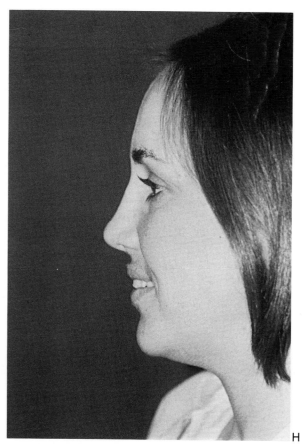

G   H

Figure 125.

FIGURE 126

Note that the postoperative views were converted to black and white from Kodachromes taken in March 1985.

Etiology: postrhinoplasty
Surgical approach: external
Surgical aims: to reduce dorsal convexity and tip projection; to correct tip asymmetry and breathing problem

Surgical Problems and Their Solution

1. Hump: leveling was completed with rasp and scalpel
2. Nasal septum
   a. Nasal obstruction corrected with a Killian submucous resection
   b. Cartilage was removed from the area of the inferior septal angle to promote subsidence of the tip in the direction of the premaxilla
3. Nasal base
   a. Scar tissue was excised to permit mobilization of the alar cartilages
   b. Both cartilages were excised at their domes
   c. The vestibular skin was dissected free from the medial ends of the lateral crura for a distance of about 5 mm
   d. Segments of cartilage were excised from remnants of the scrolls and from each lateral crus just lateral to the body to help shorten the longer leg of the basal tripod and facilitate lateral crura rotation
   e. The medial ends of the lateral crura that were in excess after rotation were trimmed appropriately
   f. A thin piece of morselized septal cartilage was used to fill a concavity at the medial end of the left lateral crus

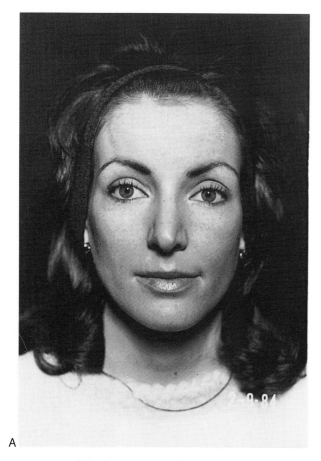

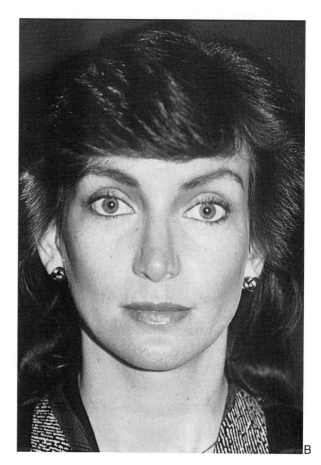

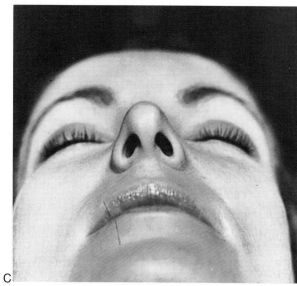

Figure 126.

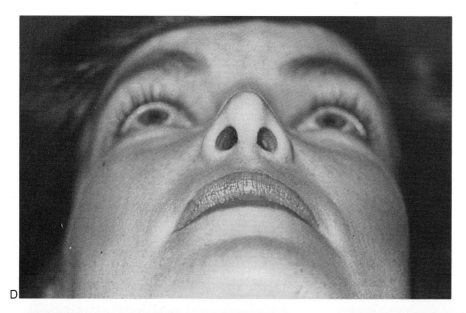

D

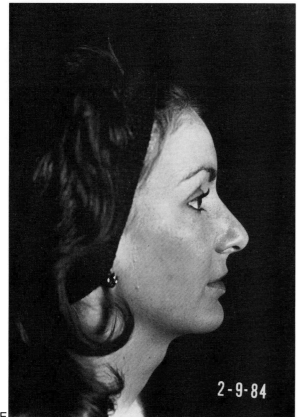

E   2-9-84

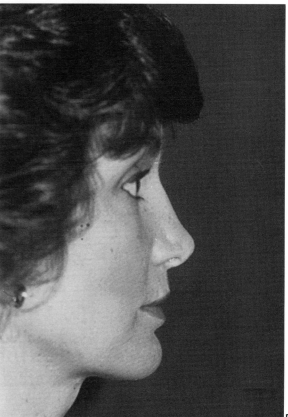

F

Figure 126.

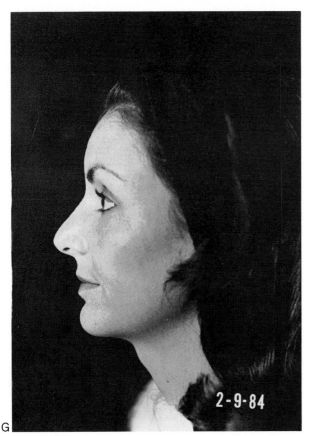

2-9-84

G

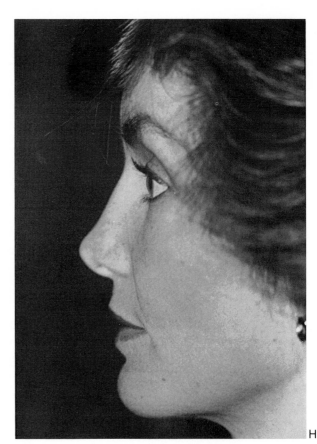

H

Figure 126.

FIGURE 127

Note that the preoperative views were taken in April 1980. Postoperative views were converted to black and white from Kodachrome transparencies taken in September 1983.

Etiology: two previous rhinoplasties
Surgical approach: external
Surgical aims: to straighten the nose; to correct supratip soft-tissue rounding; to improve lobular appearance

Surgical Problems and Their Solutions

1. Supratip soft tissue rounding: corrected by excision of hypertrophic scar tissue from the overlying skin

2. Nasal septum: submucous resection to straighten the deviated septum beneath the bony pyramid that prevented satisfactory infracture of the left wall of the bony pyramid
3. Nasal base
   a. The alar cartilages were mobilized by dissecting away the scar tissue that was binding them down
   b. The lobular asymmetry was found to be due to the fact that the cartilages had been improperly trimmed; they were equalized as well as possible
   c. An intracrural strut of autogenous septal cartilage was introduced to ensure maintenance of the desired tip projection

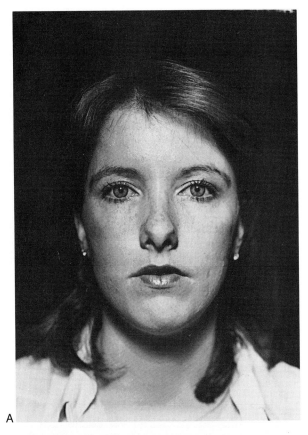

A

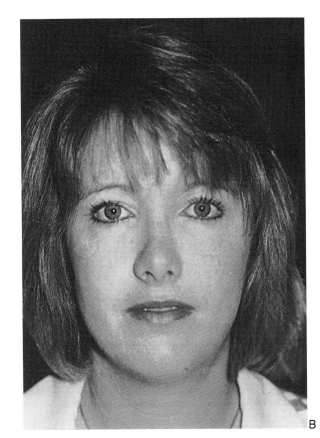

B

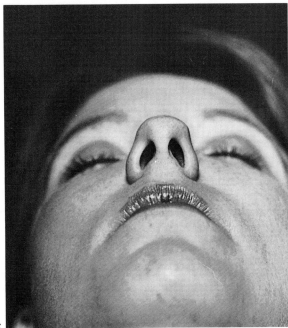

C

Figure 127.

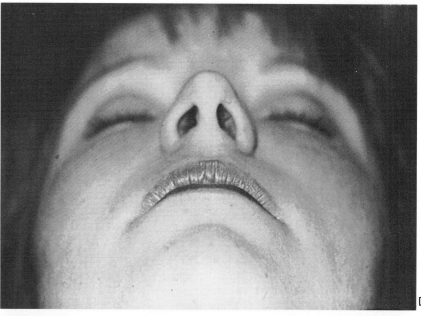

D

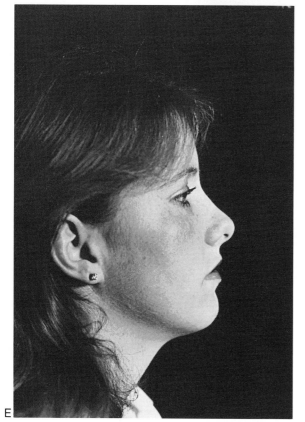

E

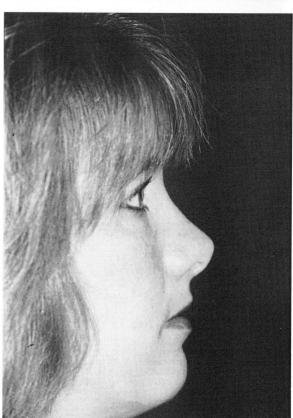

F

Figure 127.

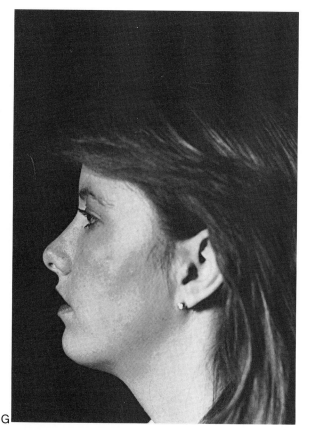
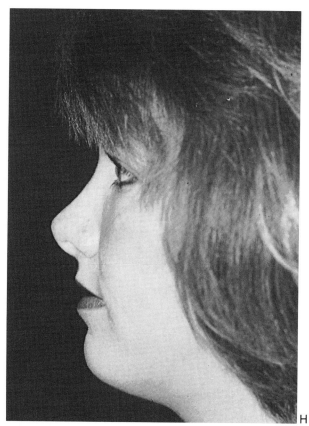

G   H

Figure 127.

FIGURE 128

Note that the preoperative photographs were taken March 1979.

Etiology: postrhinoplasty
Surgical approach: external
Surgical aims: to correct a soft tissue polly beak deformity, to narrow and increase projection of the lobule, to narrow the alae, to correct a deviated and thickened nasal septum, to narrow the bony nasal pyramid, to improve columella retraction

Surgical Problems and Their Correction

1. Correction of soft tissue polly beak deformity
   a. Dissection of hypertrophic scar tissue from the undersurface of the skin in the tip and supratip areas and over the upper lateral cartilages
   b. Crosshatching the undersurface of the dermis to improve skin pliability and drapeage
   c. Dermabrasion of the skin of the supratip area 4 months after operation
2. Reduction of lobular width: scar-tissue excision already described
3. Increased lobular projection accomplished with a septal cartilage strut inserted between the medial crura; it extended from just above the premaxillae to the apexes of the nostrils; this also lessened retraction of the nasolabial angle
4. Deviation of the quadrangular cartilage, maxillary crest, vomer, and perpendicular plate of the ethmoid corrected by classic Killian submucous resection
5. Narrowing the bony pyramid accomplished by repeat medial and lateral osteotomies after the underlying septal obstruction had been relieved
6. Alae narrowing accomplished by wedge resection from the nostril rims

Figure 128.

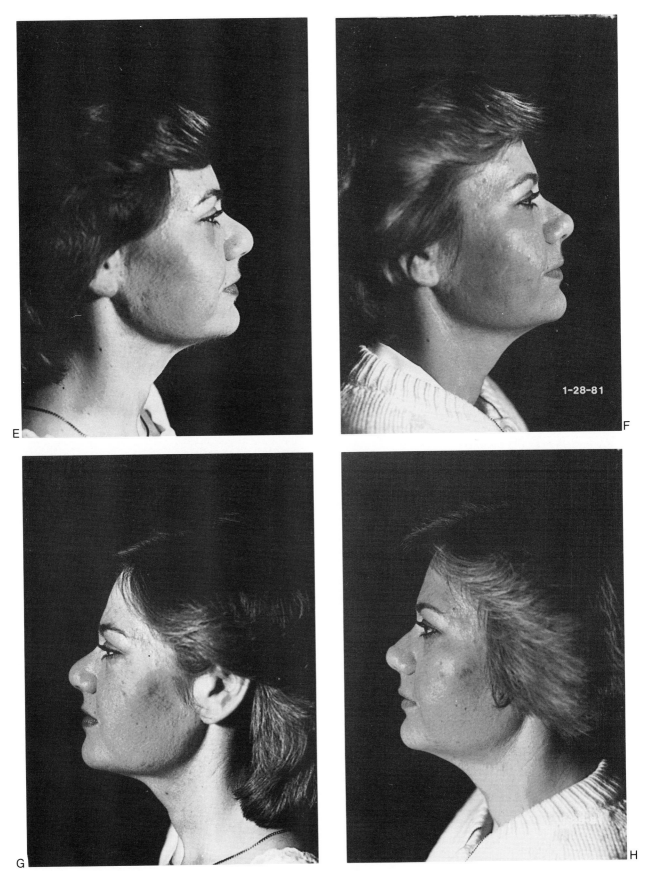

Figure 128.

FIGURE 129

Note that the postoperative views were converted to black and white from Kodachromes taken September 1985.

Etiology: three previous rhinoplasties
Surgical approach: external
Surgical aims: to correct widening of the nasal pyramid, widening and asymmetry of the lobule, columella retraction, shorten length of the nasal dorsum, repair deviation and dislocation of the remaining septal cartilage and bony septum, remove or recontour dorsal implant, and, hopefully, to improve dryness of mucous membranes and other functional problems

Surgical Problems and Their Solutions

1. Displaced solid silicone implant removed; the need for improved projection of the nasal dorsum eventually corrected by implanting two layers of morselized homogenous cartilage along the entire length of the nasal dorsum
2. Widening of the nasal pyramid improved
   a. After the twisted septum beneath the bony pyramid was straightened by submucous resection and a swinging-door procedure and morselization of the caudal septal cartilage left in situ, medial osteotomies and double lateral osteotomies were done
   b. The medial 3 mm of the upper lateral cartilages were stripped of their underlying mucosa to reduce their curvature

   c. "Returning" of the caudal ends of the upper lateral cartilages was corrected
3. Wideness, asymmetry, and poor projection of the lobule remedied
   a. Excising the scrolls of the lateral crura
   b. Cutting through the angle of each alar cartilage intramucosally, denuding the medial 5 mm of each lateral crus of its attached mucosa to reduce the curvature of the cartilage
   c. Reducing the width of the upper ends of the medial crura by 50 percent to reduce their curvature; later, they were sewn together with 4–0 polygalactin 910 sutures
   d. After the soft tissues of the premaxillary area were mobilized by undermining, a shoring strut of homogenous septal cartilage was introduced between the medial crura to help increase tip projection and correct retraction of the base of the columella; a plumping graft of morselized cartilage was inserted behind its inferior end
   e. A morselized homogenous cartilage implant was placed above the approximated medial crura and beneath the medial ends of the lateral crura to improve their projection
   f. The medial ends of the lateral crura were trimmed appropriately to achieve relative symmetry
   g. Each lateral crus was intramucosally transected lateral to the body to permit entad rotation
4. Shortening the nasal dorsum was achieved by shortening the medial ends of the lateral crura and the use of the intercrural shoring strut

NOTE: the complaint of nasal dryness and obstruction was, apparently, alleviated by straightening the septum and improving the function of the nasal valve area

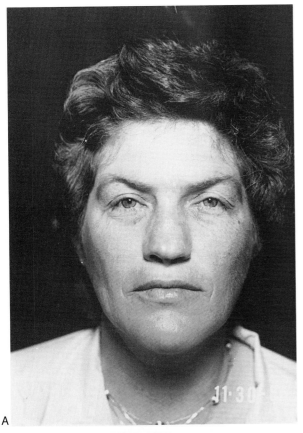

A

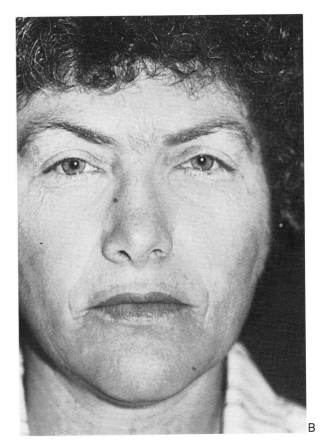

B

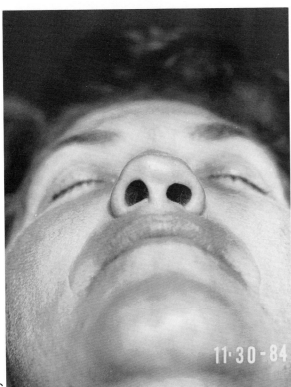

C

Figure 129.

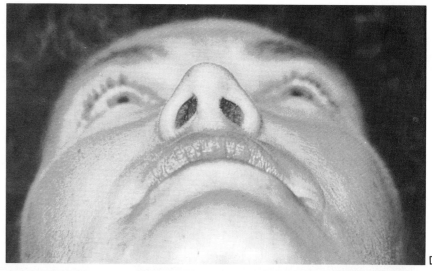

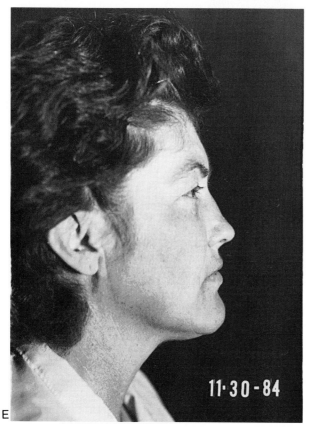

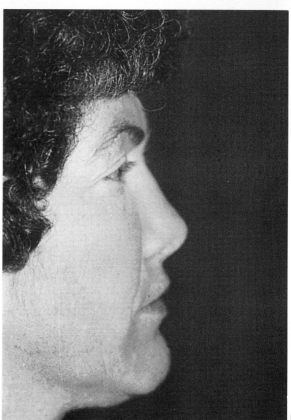

Figure 129.

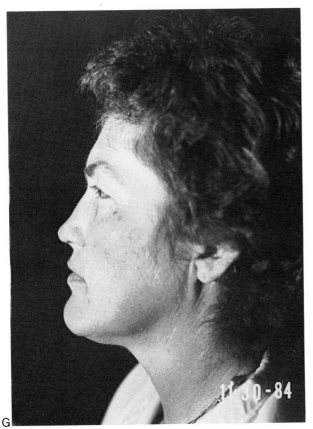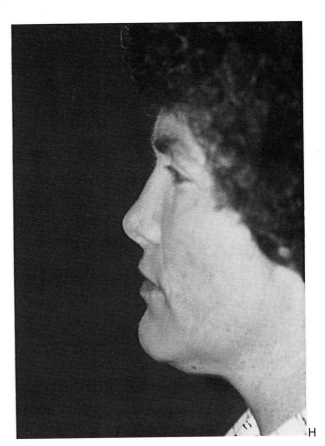

Figure 129.

REFERENCES

1. Adriani J, Zepernick R: Allergic reactions to local anesthesia. South Med J 74:694–699, 1981
2. Anderson JR: Helpful hints in nasal surgery. South Med J 56:173–176, 1963
3. Anderson JR: A new approach to rhinoplasty. Trans Am Acad Ophthalmol Otolaryngol 70:183–192, 1966
4. Anderson JR: The dynamics of rhinoplasty. Excerpta Med Int Cong Ser 206:708–710, 1969
5. Anderson JR: Straightening the crooked nose. Trans Am Acad Ophthalmol Otolaryngol 76:938–945, 1972
6. Anderson JR: Philosophical considerations in revising cosmetic surgical operations. Otolaryngol Clin North Am 7:56–64, 1974
7. Anderson JR: On the selection of patients for rhinoplasty. Otolaryngol Clin North Am 8:685–688, 1975
8. Anderson JR: A self-administered history questionnaire for cosmetic facial surgery candidates. Arch Otolaryngol 104:89–98, 1978
9. Anderson JR: A technic of rhinoplasty. In Paparella MM, Shumrick DA: Otolaryngology, 2nd ed. Philadelphia: WB, Saunders, 1980
10. Anderson JR: On planning rhinoplasty. Laryngoscope 94:1115–1116, 1984
11. Anderson JR: A reasoned approach to nasal base surgery. Arch Otolaryngol 110:349–358, June 1984
12. Anderson JR: A scale for evaluating results in rhinoplasty. Arch Otolaryngol 111:520–523, 1985
13. Anderson JR: Supratip soft-tissue rounding after rhinoplasty: Causes, prevention and treatment. Laryngoscope 86:53–56, 1976
14. Anderson JR, Johnson CM Jr, Adamson P: Open rhinoplasty: An assessment. Otolaryngol Head Neck Surg 90:272–274, 1982
15. Anderson JR, Rubin W: Retrograde intramucosal hump removal in rhinoplasty, Arch Otolaryngol 68:346–350, 1950
16. Aufricht G: Surgery of the radix and bony nose: Preliminary report of a new type of nasal clamp. Plast Reconstr Surg 22:315–321, 1958
17. Becker OJ: Principles of Otolaryngologic Plastic Surgery. Rochester, MN: American Academy of Ophthalmology and Otolaryngology, 1958
18. Becker OJ: Rhinoplasty: Cultural, esthetic and psychological aspects. Chicago Med 64:230–235, 1961
19. Beekhuis GJ: Nasal septoplasty. Otolaryngol Clin North Am 6:693–710, 1973
20. Beekhuis GJ: Nasal obstruction after rhinoplasty: Etiology and techniques for correction. Laryngoscope 86:540–547, 1976
21. Berscheid E, Walster E, Gohrnsted G: The happy American body: A survey report. Psychol Today 7:119–131, 1973
22. Bernstein L: Surgical anatomy in rhinoplasty. Otolaryngol Clin North Am 8:549–558, 1975
23. Bernstein L: Esthetics in rhinoplasty. Otolaryngol Clin North Am 8:705–715, 1975
24. Cohen S: Complications following rhinoplasty. Plast Reconstr Surg 18:213–218, 1956
25. Converse JM: Plastic Reconstructive Surgery. Philadelphia: W.B. Saunders, 1964
26. Cottle MH: Corrrective Surgery Nasal Septum and External Pyramid: Study Notes and Laboratory Manual. Chicago: American Rhinologic Society, 1960
27. Davis CL: Psychiatric screening of patients for cosmetic surgery. In Bernstein L (ed): Plastic and Reconstructive Surgery of the Head and Neck, vol I. New York: Grune & Stratton, 1981
28. Denecke HJ, Meyer R: Plastic Surgery of the Head and Neck. New York: Springer-Verlag, 1967
29. Edgerton MT, Jacobsen WE, Meyer E: Surgical-psychiatric study of patients seeking plastic (cosmetic) surgery: Ninety-eight patients with minimal deformity. Br J Plast Surg 13:136–147, 1961
30. Fairbanks DNF: Closure of nasal septal perforations. Arch Otolaryngol 106:509–513, 1980
31. Fomon S: Cosmetic Surgery, Principles and Practice. Philadelphia, J.B. Lippincott, 1960
32. Fry H: Nasal skeletal trauma and the interlocked stresses of the nasal septal cartilage. Br J Plast Surg 20:146–152, 1967
33. Gibson T, Davis WB: The distortion of autogenous cartilage grafts: Its cause and prevention. Br J Plast Surg 10:257–274, 1958
34. Goin J, Goin MK: Changing the Body: Psychological Effects of Plastic Surgery. Baltimore: Williams & Wilkins, 1981
35. Goldman IB: New technic for corrective surgery of the nasal tip. Arch Otolaryngol 58:183–187, 1953
36. Goode RL: Surgery of the incompetent nasal valve. Laryngoscope 95:546–555, 1985
37. Goodman WS: External approach to rhinoplasty. Can J Otolaryngol 2:207–210, 1973
38. Huffman WC, Lierle DM: Progress in septal surgery. Plast Reconstr Surg 20:185–198, 1957
39. Janeke JB, Wright WK: Studies on the support of the nasal tip. Arch Otolaryngol 93:458–464, 1971
40. Jennes ML: Photography in rhinoplasty. EENT Monthly 41:799–803, 1962
41. Joseph J: Nasenplastic und sontige Geischplastic. Leipzig: Curt Katitzsch, 1931
42. Lawson W, Kessler K, Biller HF: Unusual and fatal complications of rhinoplasty. Arch Otolaryngol 109:164–169, 1983
43. Liggett J: The Human Face. London: Constable, 1974
44. Macgregor FC: Transformation and Identity. New York: Quadrangle Press, 1974
45. Macgregor FC, Schaffner B: Screening patients for nasal plastic operations: Some sociologic and psychiatric considerations. Psychosom Med 12:277–291, 1950
46. Millard DR: Secondary corrective rhinoplasty. Plast Reconstr Surg 44:545–557, 1969
47. Millard DR: The versatility of a chondromucosal flap in the nasal vestibule. Plast Reconstr Surg 50:580–585, 1972
48. Pitanguy I: Surgical importance of a dermatocartilagenous ligament in bulbous noses. Plast Reconstr Surg 36:247–253, 1965
49. Powell H, Humphreys B: Proportions of the Aesthetic Face. New York: Thieme-Stratton, 1984
50. Rees TD: Aesthetic Plastic Surgery. Philadelphia: W.B. Saunders, 1980
51. Rees TD, Krupp S, Wood-Smith D: Secondary rhinoplasty. Plast Reconstr Surg 46:332–340, 1970
52. Reich J: The surgery of appearance: Psychological and related aspects. Med J Aust 2:5–13, 1969
53. Roe JO: Correction of nasal deformities by subcutaneous operations. Am Med Q 1:56–71, 1899
54. Rubin FF: Permanent change in shape of cartilage by morselization. Arch Otolaryngol 89:602–608, 1969
55. Schulman BH: Psychiatric assessment of the candidate for cosmetic surgery. Presented at the meeting of the American

Academy of Facial Plastic and Reconstructive Surgery, St. Louis, April 1973

56. Sheen JH: Achieving more nasal tip projection by use of small autogenous vomer or septal cartilage grafts. Plast Reconstr Surg 56:35–41, 1975

57. Silver AG: Pitfalls in rhinoplasty. EENT Monthly 31:556–589, 1952

58. Stucker FJ, Smith TE Jr: The nasal dorsum and cartilagenous vault: Pitfalls in management. Arch Otolaryngol 102:695–698, 1976

59. Walter C: The use of composite grafts in the head and neck region. In English G (ed): Otolaryngology. Philadelphia: Harper & Row, 1981

60. Webster RC: Advances in surgery of the tip. Otolaryngol Clin North Am 8:615–644, 1975

61. Webster RC: Revisional rhinoplasty. Otolaryngol Clin North Am 8:753–782, 1975

62. Wright MR: Self-perception of the elective surgeon and some patient perception correlates. Arch Otolaryngol 106:460–465, 1980

63. Wright MR: Management of patient dissatisfaction with results of cosmetic procedures. Arch Otolaryngol 106:466–471, 1980

64. Wright MR: How to recognize and control the problem patient. J Dermatol Surg Oncol 10:395–398, 1984

65. Wright MR, Wright WK: A psychological study of patient undergoing cosmetic surgery. Arch Otolaryngol 101:145–151, 1975

66. Wright WK: Study on hump removal in rhinoplasty. Laryngoscope 77:508–517, 1967

67. Wright WK: Surgery of the bony and cartilagenous dorsum. Otolaryngol Clin North Am 8:575–598, 1975

68. Wright WK, Kridel RWK: External septorhinoplasty: A tool for teaching and for improved results. Laryngoscope 91:945–951, 1981

Index

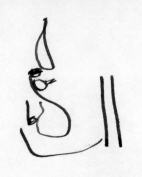